FOUR
WAY
BURN

FOUR WAY BURN

THE ALL-IN-ONE TRAINING PROGRAM FOR
STRONGER MUSCLES
MORE FLEXIBILITY
IMPROVED POSTURE AND BALANCE
INCREASED ENERGY AND POWER

RALF HENNIG CPT, CCS, CCES
FOREWORD BY BILL CLINTON

RODALE

© 2007 by Ralf Hennig
Foreword © 2007 by Bill Clinton

Rodale books may be purchased for business or promotional use or for special sales. For information, please
write to: Special Markets Department, Rodale Inc., 733 Third Avenue, New York, NY 10017.

Printed in the United States of America
Rodale Inc. makes every effort to use acid-free ♾, recycled paper ♻

Photographs by Mitch Mandel
Book design by Tara Long

Library of Congress Cataloging-in-Publication Data

Hennig, Ralf.
    Four way burn : the all-in-one training program for stronger muscles, more flexibility, improved posture
and balance, increased energy and power / Ralf Hennig ; foreword by Bill Clinton.
        p.   cm.
    Includes index.
    ISBN–13 978–1–59486–543–5 paperback
    ISBN–10 1–59486–543–4 paperback
    1. Physical fitness.   2. Exercise.   3. Vitality.   I. Title.
RA781.H4644 2009
613.7'1—dc22   2006036695

Distributed to the trade by Holtzbrinck Publishers

2   4   6   8   10   9   7   5   3   1   paperback

RODALE
LIVE YOUR WHOLE LIFE™

We inspire and enable people to improve their lives and the world around them
For more of our products visit **rodalestore.com** or call 800-848-4735

I dedicate this book to all the people whose goal is a pain-free and independent lifestyle.

And I dedicate this book to all the healthcare professionals who are helping people to achieve this goal.

I also dedicate this book to the athletic population and coaches, whose goal is to perform at their best.

Be responsible.

Contents

Foreword by Bill Clinton ix

Acknowledgments xi

Introduction xiii

PART 1

Four Way Burn: Conditioning for Life

Chapter 1: A Balanced Approach to Wellness and Fitness 3

Chapter 2: *Four Way Burn* Will Change Your Life 15

PART 2

Progressive Cycles Move You to Success

Chapter 3: The First Cycle 27

Chapter 4: The Second Cycle 45

Chapter 5: The Third Cycle 58

Chapter 6: The Fourth Cycle 70

PART 3

Adapting *Four Way Burn* for Your Needs

Chapter 7: Stay On Track While You're Traveling 87

Chapter 8: Lose Weight with *Four Way Burn* 105

Chapter 9: The Right Moves Can Bring Back Your Strong, Flexible Back 117

PART 4

Using *Four Way Burn* for Peak Sports Performance

Chapter 10: Get Ready for Walking and Running with *Four Way Burn* 147

Chapter 11: Good Form Keeps a Cyclist's Body Rolling Along 174

Chapter 12: Golf: Complex Moves Require Thorough Conditioning...........................199

Chapter 13: Increase Control and Power on the Tennis Court...................................226

Appendix 247

Index..257

Foreword

By Bill Clinton

I started working with Ralf Hennig about 5 years ago. At the time I thought I was in pretty good shape, just a few pounds overweight. Ralf told me he wanted to work on my strength, balance, and flexibility and said the weight loss would come if I watched my diet. He said we would do some light weight work with a lot of repetitions but most of the time we would be working on flexibility, building balance and strength in all muscle groups.

In the first session, I learned that in spite of years of jogging, golfing, and other physical activity, I was weak, inflexible, and unbalanced. The drills he put me through showed where the problems were, and as I learned to do them, I could see and feel the difference in a short time. My strength and flexibility increased, and my posture improved. But the biggest improvement came in my balance, an area in which I had always had difficulty. I didn't ride a bicycle until I was 22, or water-ski for a few years after that. When I tried to snow-ski, I injured my knee so badly I was disabled for 3 months. Now I can do all sorts of stretch and balance drills on one leg. In my 60th year, this is of great practical importance. The winters are long in New York. In each of the last three, I have slipped on the ice, but I didn't fall once thanks to the sense of balance and recovery I developed doing Ralf's drills. Sixty-year-old broken bones take a long time to heal. Thanks to Ralf, it's one physical challenge I've avoided so far.

Many of the movements in this book look very simple. Some of them are. But if you do them properly, you will find them challenging and helpful. They are designed to allow you to begin them at any age or fitness level, then to increase the repetitions and difficulty as you are able.

The routines can be done with a light medicine ball, or a beach ball with light weights that strap onto wrists or ankles. However, I recommend you get the Performance Ball Ralf designed, because it's the right weight and its soft texture aids in the development of grip and forearm strength and in balance.

The key to success with this program is to be persistent but not impatient. Do it three to five times a week, and you'll be amazed at how much better you'll look and feel.

Acknowledgments

To my parents, who taught me to be generous, to have integrity, and to be honest. In the midst of their tedious and neverending work, they made the time to teach me qualities such as courage, racial tolerance, discipline, a strong work ethic, politeness, punctuality, and respect, simply by practicing these principles themselves. These important guidelines helped me to develop my self-worth.

To my children, Liesl and William (Wilhelm), who give me laughter every day . . . and sometimes high blood pressure, too. Reflecting often on their carefree and expanding lives has given me the strength to keep growing.

To my siblings Mario, Christine, and Angelika. I have realized that without siblings, the world is smaller.

To president Bill Clinton and Senator Hillary Clinton. They have shown me that they are not just talking about the need for better health in America, but they're also practicing preventive health care themselves. Despite the intense weekly schedule that each of them maintains, they are making the time to stay healthy and fit to perform at their highest levels. The health care of our nation is very important to each of them.

To all the clients who trusted me. And special thanks to the ones who took extra time to share their testimonies and let me use them in this book.

To Rodale, my publisher, who shares my vision for self-reliance. And thanks to their professional staff, in particular, editor Amy Super, who recognized the unique *Four Way Burn* concept and bridged my interest as the author with her publisher's goal of creating a long-lasting book.

To Eric, who helped me put my German-American writing into proper English. I wanted my explanations to be clear and straightforward so they'd easily make sense to the readers.

Special thanks to Richard Miller.

And to Stavros. A true friend. You gave me a kick in the butt just in time. . . .

For Phil. Rest in peace.

Introduction

Science has proven that our bodies are meant to move. Without movement, our bodies deteriorate. That's simply how humankind has evolved.

We have bones for support, joints to let us bend in many directions, muscles to put us into motion, and a brain and nervous system to direct it all.

All these parts are well designed and carefully assembled. We have them so that we can *move*, not sit still.

Unfortunately, for many people, this precious ability is slowly disappearing. Too many people are developing weakness, stiffness, and pain because they're simply not moving enough. Too much sitting around year after year will cause your muscles and joints to atrophy and weaken.

Other people lose their ability to keep moving because they're not approaching their physical activities in a healthy manner. Overusing your body by doing the same motions day after day without variety can result in imbalance and injury. And too much exercise, without the proper amount of sleep and a balanced intake of nutrients, will also cause the body to break down. You need time to recover, rebuild, and grow, and this process occurs while you sleep at night.

Either way, you can lose your strength, flexibility, and aerobic capacity very gradually, so initially you don't realize these components of fitness are dwindling. These abilities leave us in tiny increments, and we adjust to them at first by limiting our activities. Our ability to move with total freedom becomes more reduced over time, and we lose the confidence that we can do the things we used to do.

You may be able to ignore the stiffness and aches in your muscles and joints at first. You might make adjustments to your life to cope with the discomfort. Maybe you stop playing tennis, even though you love the game. Maybe you have to hire a cleaning person because you can't bend or squat down because of pain in your hips, back, or knees. Some people even sell their homes and buy a single-story house so they don't have to climb stairs.

Pain is what I call the last indicator that a part of your body has been deteriorating for some time, perhaps over many years. If you don't maintain your strength so that you can carry your own body's weight, and if you don't work to preserve your flexibility so that you can reach, bend, twist, and move through your basic daily functions, you will suffer the consequences someday. It may take years, but ignoring your body's basic fitness needs will lead to breakdown. Before you start learning about the *Four Way Burn* program, remember: People die a slow death by sitting or lying down too much.

Fortunately, you *can* prevent stiffness, aches, and pains. Even if your movements have already become limited, you can regain your strength and flexibility.

But keeping your body in good working condition takes a regular commitment. This book will teach you how to do it.

I didn't write this book to just introduce another short-lived wellness or fitness trend, but rather to demonstrate that all people—male or female, young or old—can change their lifestyles to improve and maintain their wellness, fitness, and physical performance no matter what physical shape they're in now.

Plenty of books are already available that teach you how to improve your aerobic fitness, your strength, or your flexibility. Other books can teach you about anatomy and how to rehabilitate your body after injuries. In addition, your doctor can tell you what you can do to improve your health. A physical therapist can tell you how to help your body recover from an injury so that it can work properly again.

But existing books don't put all these aspects of fitness together so that you can improve them all in a balanced way. And doctors and physical therapists aren't coordinating their skills well with preventive healthcare professionals to benefit the public.

Four Way Burn is the first book that brings *all* this knowledge together in one program. With one simple piece of equipment—a weighted ball—you can improve your strength, flexibility, and aerobic fitness all at the same time, so these components of your fitness stay balanced. At the same time, the simple techniques in this program will provide physical rehabilitation for your body so you can keep it working well and avoid injuries before they ever happen.

This book will also show you how to use a body part that most exercise books leave out: your brain. Being physically fit requires more than just the body. In reality, performing well requires an interaction between the mind and the body, because without the mind guiding our movements, our bodies will not move. To attain long and lasting fitness, what you really need is a conditioning program that works your mind and body together.

I've worked in the fitness industry for 25 years, and in that time I've trained top athletes and people working to leave their wheelchairs. I've worked with corporate CEOs who could afford to bring in any personal trainer they wanted, and I've led group fitness classes in my small town.

I've learned that our bodies all work the same way, more or less, and we all need to follow the same rules for healthy living.

The conditioning program I have designed—and used with clients for many years—can help *all* people stay healthy and fit so that they can better perform their lifestyle activities or regain the health and fitness they once had.

Before we get to the actual program, I'd like to take a moment to explain how I became involved in the fitness industry. During years of enjoying many types of physical activities, I've traveled thousands of miles and devoted countless hours to physical conditioning. The result: this book, *Four Way Burn*.

THE ORIGINS OF *FOUR WAY BURN*

I've always watched developments in the fitness industry carefully so that I could use the best ones with my clients and discard the ones that weren't going to pan out.

I keep my shelves filled with exercise physiology textbooks and journals so that I can catch improvements long before they come to the attention of the public. I've worked in physical rehabilitation and professional sports training, and I've added the best that each has to offer to my repertoire. I've thrown myself into all sorts of physical activities so I can personally learn how the body responds to different types of movement.

And not to brag too much, but I can also cook an excellent Wiener schnitzel.

The varied career path I've taken has allowed me to pick up many skills and experiences and mold them into what I feel is the best fitness program you can find.

My career started far away in Germany, where I took my father's advice and began training to be a chef when I was a teenager. He wanted me to have a job where I would always have enough to eat, since he grew up in a time of scarce food. I, however, was more interested in being able to travel and participate in sports that weren't available in Germany.

After I completed my culinary training, yet was still in my teens, I moved to a seasonal hotel in Switzerland that was situated about 10,000 feet high in the mountains. Visitors came for the skiing, of course, but also for hang-gliding and parachuting off cliffs. It became a hot spot for young athletes. Working as a chef requires long hours, but I made the most of my free time by skiing and engaging in other athletic pursuits as much as possible.

Once I'd refined my skiing skills—and gotten my fill of the cold—it was time for a different sport. I was ready to try scuba diving and windsurfing. So I headed off to Saudi Arabia, where a new hotel was looking for upcoming, innovative chefs to bring European cuisine to the region. When I wasn't in the restaurant kitchen, I was windsurfing on the Red Sea and scuba diving under it. I also started traveling to Malaysia, where I began learning shotokan karate and kung fu.

I was a busy young man. But my life was about to become far busier. My next stop was the Cayman Islands, where I took a job as the head chef in a restaurant. I got the chance to refine my skills with seafood, but my attention became more and more focused on fitness. The martial arts were very popular in the islands, and I began competing in kickboxing and other styles of martial arts, still continuing to train under some of the world's top instructors.

I began teaching aerobics classes in the mornings at a workout facility before heading off to dive and practice karate in the afternoons, then cooking at the restaurant from the evening until late at night. I led classes in kickboxing aerobics long before the activity became popular, and we stepped up and down on benches and chairs before anyone had heard of step aerobics.

When I flew off to a new location or went home to see my family, I often flew through New York. In those days, everyone traveling through New York wanted to stay there, and my next stop was Long Island. There I started picking up more skills and experience as a fitness instructor.

I worked for fitness legend Jack La Lanne in his workout facility. At the time, high-impact aerobics were popular, and I enjoyed teaching the classes. I was known as the strict German guy—I didn't allow gum, water bottles, or talking. The students loved it, but because we drilled repetitive motions and didn't emphasize proper form, injuries were common.

I went on to open my own restaurants north of the city, but I always taught fitness during the day. After years of running myself ragged, I finally decided that I needed to channel all my energy into one field and be extra good at one thing. I went with my passion, which was fitness, and I have never looked back.

I settled down an hour north of New York City, became an American citizen, and threw myself completely into helping people make their bodies stronger. I worked for a time as a trainer at a sports program run by tennis star Ivan Lendl, where I helped athletes balance their bodies and protect themselves from the injuries that are common to tennis players. For more than a decade, I've owned my own personal training company. I've helped people with spinal cord injuries regain strength so they could leave their wheelchairs, and I've also designed fitness programs for a children's camp.

But I spend most of my time teaching fitness classes and working with individuals. Many of my clients are heads of corporations and movers and shakers on Wall Street. One of my clients is a former president of the United States. His wife, a senator, is another client. Most of the people I work with can afford the absolute best personal training, and they're hard-driving individuals who demand results. They feel that my program gives them everything they need from a workout in a short period of time.

I'm experienced enough in many sports to know what types of development each activity requires and how each type of sport can cause specific injuries. I run and bicycle long-distance every week, and I ski and practice indoor rock climbing regularly. My high level of training in several forms of martial arts has taught me how to move the body with grace, power, and efficiency while maximizing agility and balance.

I've spent a lot of time figuring out what concept and what tool are best for my clients to strengthen and condition their musculoskeletal systems and to reinforce all the other functional skills that are needed daily.

In my method, mind and body work in harmony to achieve total fitness. Through specially designed drills, you challenge and train your muscles and nervous system proportionally and at the same time. Conditioning the mind and body at the same time will enable you to better handle whatever activity comes your way.

I've practiced the program in this book myself for many years to keep fit, and it's helped hundreds of clients use their bodies better, too. I traveled all over the globe to gather the skills that I put into it. And now I offer it to you.

CONDITIONING FOR LIFE

With my program, those of you who are tight or stiff can lengthen your muscles and make your joints more flexible. Those of you who are more flexible and want to be stronger can improve your strength. If you're already athletic, you will be better prepared for the sport of your choice and lower your risk of overuse injuries.

If you just don't feel well and you're ready to get healthy, *Four Way Burn* will give you the tools you need to live a healthy, self-reliant life. It's not too late. You can relearn how to move properly and consistently, which will rebuild your body and improve it.

Once you feel healthier, you'll be ready to challenge your physical fitness levels past the boundaries you have established. Every year, athletes set new records. You have the same fundamental physical makeup as an athlete, and you can set and achieve goals of your own if you pursue them in a balanced way. Challenge yourself to meet your goals, even if they're as simple as being able to do your daily chores with less stiffness and pain, or conditioning your body so you can shed extra pounds. You can do it.

I designed this program to move you through increasingly challenging activities. It starts off easily—so you don't have to plunge into a program that's difficult and hard to learn.

And it provides you with the right amount of strength and flexibility, as well as all the other important fundamental functional skills you need. You don't have to worry about following one program for strength, another for aerobic conditioning, and another for flexibility. They're all here in one simple program.

While holding a weighted ball, you'll perform movements that require coordination and careful mental focus. At your own pace, you'll reconnect your body parts and your mind so that they communicate better with each other and so that you can control them with more ease. This program uses a weighted ball because it's so versatile, handy, and fun to use. Because you've played with a ball many times in your life, you're less likely to feel intimidated by this piece of equipment than you would a weight-lifting machine. The ball invites you to play and challenge yourself.

You'll also develop the left and right sides of your body equally. Over the years, because you use your right or left arm more frequently, you've developed imbalances that can cause weaknesses and injuries due to overuse or lack of use. Once you start moving much more easily, you'll probably realize that your body hasn't been properly balanced in a long time.

Your many body parts are united into a chain. If one link of the chain breaks down and the weak link is not addressed, soon other links will follow. As the saying goes, "The body is only as strong as the weakest link." In today's culture, which encourages us to live sedentary lifestyles, you must maintain a regular fitness training program to stay healthy and keep moving with full freedom.

You're the one who can reap the rewards of better fitness—but you're also the one who first must make the investment of consistent daily physical activity. No one else can manage your wellness and fitness better than you can.

I am convinced you will succeed.

FOUR WAY BURN:
CONDITIONING
FOR LIFE

1

A BALANCED APPROACH TO WELLNESS AND FITNESS

When it comes to fitness, America has become a land of extremes. At one extreme you'll find millions of Americans who don't want to be physically active. On the other end are the many Americans who enjoy staying active—but who subject their bodies to a lot of wear and tear due to the way they move.

Both of these attitudes cause a lot of avoidable illness and injuries. But let's start with the more common problem: people who don't move enough.

NOT WANTING TO MOVE LEADS TO NOT *BEING ABLE* TO MOVE

More than half of Americans don't do *any* vigorous activity in their leisure time. Think about that—most people don't move without stopping for even 10 minutes a week! Only a small portion of the population—24 percent—will get up and do vigorous activity three times a week or more.

Our bodies are meant to move a lot. We're supposed to be running, walking, jumping, lifting, turning, and reaching every single day. But too few people enjoy making the effort to put their bodies through these motions. (By the way, I should tell you this now: I don't like the word *exercise*. That sounds like a chore. I like to say *physical activity* or *movement*. That sounds more fun and exciting.)

Most of us don't work in jobs that require much physical exertion, either. Compared to previous generations, not many people do farm work, chop down trees, or have demanding factory jobs that require bodily effort. Instead, too many jobs nowadays require us to sit. We type on computers, send voicemails, talk on the phone, and drive around to see clients.

Keeping a household running doesn't require much effort, either. Most of us have washers and dryers in our own homes, so we don't have to carry heavy baskets of clothes back and forth to the Laundromat. We have dishwashers that clean our pots and pans to save us from even that minor exertion.

Most of us live in cities and towns that require us to hop in our cars and drive to the store instead of walking or cycling. Once there, we look for the closest parking space so we don't have to walk a few extra feet. Most supermarkets and department stores now keep a fleet of electric carts in the lobby for the many customers who are too unfit or unable to walk while shopping.

In short, if we don't want to move much, we don't have to do so. Why move when a machine will move for you? Why even leave the house to see a movie or eat a meal if you can order anything you want by phone or over the Internet? Many people find it "freeing" to not have to do extra work.

Actually, though, these conveniences aren't freeing. They're just the opposite. They *rob* you of your freedom. Being well means you're free from sickness and injury. Having full use of your body means you're free of limitations. You must keep moving if you want to be fit. You must be fit if you want to be well. This idea is key to my philosophy as a fitness professional: *Movement is a basic principle that's required if you want to enjoy wellness.*

Movement keeps your musculoskeletal system strong. It keeps your heart and lungs working like they should. When you keep moving, your blood pumps properly, your body's countless chemicals stay more balanced, and your body and mind feel *good.*

When you don't move, your body starts breaking down. It can deteriorate so slowly that you don't even notice it. The majority of Americans are now overweight or obese, and the number keeps rising. More than 180,000 people will die this year from cancer that could have been prevented with better nutrition, more physical activity, and maintenance of a healthy weight. And many cases of heart disease, the number one killer in America, can be prevented with a more active lifestyle.

In other words, the equivalent of the population of a big city dies early *every single year* in part because people don't stay fit.

But being out of shape reduces the quality of your life, too. When you remain seated or lying down day after day, you develop neck and back pain as your spine and shoulders become unbalanced. Your muscles grow weak. Your heart and lungs become unaccustomed to challenge. When the moment comes that you want to get up and play with your kids or do a heavy chore, you can't do it! When I see parents with their kids at the park, the kids are playing and the parents are often sitting on a bench, unwilling or unable to run and jump or throw a ball.

Your mind suffers when you're not moving around enough. When you're sedentary, you're more likely to feel depressed. You don't feel good about yourself. Your stress builds up and you have no healthy outlet to release it.

In short, when you don't move enough, you're not "free" at all. You become stuck in a body that no longer works properly. Carrying extra weight around your midsection pulls your back out of alignment. Sitting at a computer keyboard all day causes you to hunch over, putting a strain on your neck and shoulders. You're out of breath when you trot a few hundred feet or lift a heavy load, and your elbows and shoulders hurt after a few minutes of painting or yard work.

Being unhealthy through lack of movement is one of the two extremes you'll see when you look at the fitness of the average American. At the other end of the scale, you'll find people who try to stay fit but hurt their bodies from moving the *wrong* ways.

Can *Four Way Burn* Help Me?

If you have to answer yes to any of the following statements, *Four Way Burn* can help you gain greater control over your body and participate in activities with more vitality and flexibility:

- ▶ I have bad balance.
- ▶ When I'm at parties or functions, I need to sit down.
- ▶ My feet hurt, or I've sprained my ankles on more than one occasion.
- ▶ I can't stand on one leg for more than a minute.
- ▶ I have chronic stiffness in my knees and fingers.
- ▶ I have shoulder problems or nagging pain between my shoulder blades.
- ▶ I have hip pain.
- ▶ I've pulled a groin muscle before.
- ▶ I have trouble opening a can due to my weak grip.
- ▶ I've spent a lot of time carrying a child on one hip.
- ▶ I'm a professional or recreational athlete.

ALL PHYSICAL ACTIVITIES DEMAND PROPER STRENGTH AND FLEXIBILITY

Look at weekend warriors. These people want to resume playing basketball but haven't played hard in 10 years. They know they've done it well before, but they can't understand why they get hurt when they start again. I frequently see guys returning to the soccer field after they haven't played in a long time. They put their cleats back on and run, and what happens? They get sprained ankles. There's no good reason for an ankle to become sprained. But over time, its strength and flexibility can deteriorate.

A friend and colleague of mine, Evan Karas, MD, an orthopedic surgeon at the Mount Kisco Medical Group in New York, treats these injuries all of the time. He says, "What I see a lot is people who have been sedentary for a long time who get very enthusiastic all of a sudden about working out, but they don't go about it the proper way. They start doing very stressful activities quickly and they ramp up too quickly, and they start getting overuse injuries and their bodies start to break down."

Tennis, basketball, and other sports require more strength, flexibility, and balance than you need in your everyday life. When playing these sports causes injuries, you realize that your body has gradually been losing its abilities.

As you grow older, your tendons, which anchor muscles to bone in your joints, become more brittle and can't handle the stress that they could handle when you were younger, Dr. Karas says. "The whole concept of dynamic fitness, which is strengthening muscle groups around a particular body region to take stress off it, becomes more important as the tendons that are moving the skeleton become more brittle."

Even people who are constantly physically active are at risk of injury. The people who are always out running and biking can cause overuse injuries in their muscles and joints from repetitive motion. People who want to get better at running—perhaps to train for a marathon or other race—often think they must keep drilling their bodies harder and harder. They simply run more, going faster and farther.

Overtraining doesn't make you better, though. In reality, your musculoskeletal system can only do so much of a given motion before it breaks down. When you run again and again, you *over*develop certain parts of your body while others become *under*developed. Your body gets out of balance, your joints start moving improperly, and all that running starts to cause damage.

The same thing happens with cyclists. Many people start bicycling because their knees or hips are hurt from running. These people often think that to become better cyclists they need to spend more time on a bike. But you can only ride a bicycle a certain amount, too. Cycling doesn't impact you the way running does, but it does put a lot of stress on your hips, knees, and back.

I could go on and on: Tennis players think they must play more tennis to get their bodies to perform better on the court. Golfers think they have to tee up and swing more to get conditioned for golfing.

It's just not true. Overdoing specific motions simply causes you to get hurt. You get knee and hip pain from running too far. Your elbow or shoulder starts hurting when you return a serve. Your lower back aches from driving golf balls.

It's no wonder that musculoskeletal conditions are the leading cause of activity limitations for American adults, and that the number of physical therapists is rising because so many people need help getting their bodies to work properly again.

Most people simply don't require their bodies to stay physically active, so they lose the ability to function well. And the people who *do* stay physically active often break their bodies down by using them too much in the wrong manner.

FINALLY—A CONDITIONING PROGRAM THAT MEETS *ALL* YOUR NEEDS

The *Four Way Burn* program is designed to help both types of people bring their bodies into balance and improve their physical function. Maybe you've never enjoyed "exercise" because it doesn't fit within your lifestyle. Perhaps doing situps, curling a barbell, or running on a treadmill felt like too much work just to build skills that aren't really useful to you.

This program is totally different. I know—you've heard that many times before. But *Four Way Burn* really is a new approach to fitness. I don't want you to build big muscles. I don't want you to focus only on your speed or your endurance. I don't even want you to think of this as a weight-loss program, although it can play a vital role in helping you lose weight if you wish to do so.

Instead, I want this program to give you a comprehensive and complete workout in less time than you'd need to devote to other types of exercise. During one session, you'll be improving your strength, flexibility, agility, and coordination, from fingertips to toes. You're not lifting weights on one day, doing aerobics the next, and straining through periodic stretching sessions. *You get all these benefits at one time.*

You'll strengthen your joints and work each body part in its proper proportion using real-world motions. You won't just move a body part up and down or back and forth, because your body doesn't move in these lateral motions in real life. Instead, as in daily life, this program will move your body in many planes, with the many parts working together as a team.

This program will help you create a "buffer zone," an extra level of fitness that gives you the capacity to maneuver and carry the loads you need to lift during the day. With *Four Way Burn*, you'll be better able to carry briefcases, suitcases, boxes, and bags of groceries. You'll be able to bend over and pick things up without hurting your back, and you'll be able to walk without growing winded. You'll be ready to scoop up a running toddler with one arm and open a door with the other. You'll get in and out of your car without stiffness and discomfort. You'll improve your posture and have less neck pain, headaches, and stiffness while working at a computer.

I want you to be able to do things you may not have done for a long time, or even things you never thought you could do.

I've created a regular program—which forms the central part of this book—for anyone who just wants to stay fit. But I've also included special programs later in the book that you can do if you're an avid jogger, cyclist, golfer, or tennis player. By adding a few *Four Way Burn* sessions to your weekly activities, you'll keep your body balanced and resistant to injury. Your posture and alignment will improve. Muscles that have grown tight will relax, improving your body mechanics. Your nondominant hand and arm will grow more proficient, since this program works both sides of your body equally.

A bicyclist will be stronger on climbs.

A runner will have longer and more powerful strides.

A tennis player will have fewer knee, lower back, and ankle problems.

A golfer will hit consistently longer drives and be more precise on putts.

People who play other sports will jump, turn, squat, and sprint with more power and control.

In addition, I've created a version of the *Four Way Burn* program specifically for people with a history of back problems. If you've had trouble with your back, do this program, which is described in Chapter 9, before you do the main program in this book. The special back program will give you the strength and flexibility you need in order to enjoy the main *Four Way Burn* moves.

America's overall health is currently in crisis. Too often we ignore our bodies' needs, and we only worry about physical problems once they've arisen. But even the best doctor or most skilled physical therapist can only do so much to make you healthy again. *You're* in the best position to truly keep yourself fit and healthy.

Your body absolutely craves the kinds of movement that this program offers. By balancing your musculoskeletal system and going through your full range of movements at each workout, you will give your body what it needs. You'll find that you stay *free* from illness and injury. You'll be *free* to enjoy more activities.

You'll discover that fitness isn't a chore. It's the key to enjoying a fuller, happier life.

Sanford Weill

Even if you've risen to the top of the business world (and a major medical college is named in your honor), you still need to provide your body with a variety of physical activities to keep it working properly.

Just ask Sanford Weill, the chairman emeritus of Citigroup, who has been doing the *Four Way Burn* techniques to improve his fitness for several years.

When he was looking for someone to help him live a healthier life, "to be perfectly honest, I didn't know what I was looking for, except a trainer," he says. "What I found was somebody who is incredibly dedicated to creating a better way of life, and who is evangelical about your weight and conditioning and how you conduct your whole life, rather than just the hour you're working with him."

Now, when he wakes up in the morning, he thinks about what types of aerobic activities he'll do during the day, such as walking. When he sits down at a restaurant, he applies what he's learned about how to eat in a healthy manner.

He retired in 2006 as CEO of Citigroup—a global financial services company—and is now applying his energy and vigor to philanthropy, travel, and other pursuits. His wife, Joan, who also works with me, also remains "very fit," he says.

At 73, he says, "I think the need for discipline is greater. I think that it's important that I stay fit, because some of the functions do get a little bit worn out, and I have to be in better shape to maintain the abilities that you have as a younger person."

With his love of fitness and helping others, Sandy might just make a good personal trainer himself if he ever needed another challenge someday.

"It's great to have a profession that creates an income while doing good for people. When clients feel better physically, they then feel better about themselves and can also do more good," he says.

MANY TYPES OF EXERCISE LEAD TO IMBALANCE

I've closely watched the fitness field evolve and change over the past 20 years, and I've noticed that many of the trends in fitness come from the worlds of physical therapy and professional athletic training. These include devices such as:

- ▶ Foam roller tubes that you lie upon to massage your muscles and improve your balance
- ▶ Rubber tubing that you pull and stretch to improve your strength
- ▶ Inflatable Swiss balls for improving your balance and strengthening core muscles
- ▶ Slide boards, which allow you to slide from side to side while you wear slick booties
- ▶ Recumbent bikes, which allow you to recline while you work the pedals

The list goes on and on. However, just because these developments were devised by experts doesn't mean that using them to train individual body parts is good for you.

I have explored *all* the methods and tools to improve your fitness and performance, and I've used many of them with clients. However, many of these methods were short-lived since they created either too much muscle tightness or too much joint looseness. I came to the realization that there was often something missing that kept these tools and techniques from being complete.

To learn how the body works, and how fitness trends can take the wrong approach, let's first consider a person who injures her wrist and requires physical therapy. First she lets her wrist rest to help it heal from the initial injury. That means she's not just resting her wrist, but also her upper arm and the shoulder girdle, which includes muscles throughout her shoulder and upper back that keep the shoulder in place. All these muscles begin to atrophy.

Ideally the physical therapist will help this patient strengthen her wrist *and* her upper arm and shoulder. So the patient needs to not just repair her injured wrist, but reintegrate it back into an arm and shoulder that are proportionally strong and flexible. If she fixes only her wrist and not the rest of her arm and shoulder—which have also been out of commission— her body becomes unbalanced and at risk for injury.

When you use a trendy device as the sole focus of your workout, you can develop similar problems. Take the stretch bands and tubing that are used for strength training. They require you to stretch out and back in a straight line. You go out and back, out and back, over and over, using relatively few muscles.

However, in real life, your body doesn't move in a linear fashion. You don't move in straight lines forward or side-to-side. You don't move your arms and legs in simple up-and-down movements. You move in different planes. You move in angles. You lean down to pick up a bag, stand up and twist to put it on a counter. You use big muscles in your arms, legs, and core, and many smaller muscles that support them.

Let's move on to another example. Consider how a professional sports team trains. I'm picturing a soccer team, since I grew up in Europe, but a basketball or football team works well in this analogy, too. A smart coach requires team members to hone their important individual skills, but they spend a lot of time working together, too. Just like your muscles, each player has a specialty, but they must also seamlessly work together. They act as one unit, passing the ball back and forth and understanding where the other players are going to go.

When you use weights to train your body, you run the risk of overdeveloping individual parts so that they don't work smoothly together. When you sit down at a weight machine, you get into a fixed position dictated by the machine—not necessarily the best position for your body. Each of us has different-sized legs or arms, different histories, and different amounts of wear and tear from the next person. But machines don't know that.

So you sit down at a machine to do curls to strengthen your biceps, and you probably set it on a heavy weight so you'll gain more strength quickly. Over time, your biceps will get strong. But if you don't also appropriately strengthen your rear shoulder girdle, which includes muscles in your back, it can't hold the new load of your heavier arms in the right place. You develop bad posture because you have trouble holding your arms the proper way. Eventually you're going to have neck, shoulder, or rotator cuff problems if you keep moving in the same imbalanced manner.

In addition, when you use heavy weights, the load overwhelms your normal movements. You're limited in how you can move, and your natural pace slows down. Being able to use your normal pace while working out is an important aspect of functional fitness.

Also, when you create big muscles with heavy weights, you have to work hard to maintain them. The more muscle mass you put on, the more you have to work to keep it. It's very hard work, it's not fun, and you can get burned out very quickly. You may drop out periodically, and when you start again you have to use lighter weights or you'll be injured.

Don't get me wrong: Strength is important. However, you also need flexibility. When you're simply lifting weights, 100 percent of your effort is going into lifting that load, and you can't spare any more energy or focus on other important functional skills that are necessary for total fitness, including flexibility.

Without flexibility, you lose the freedom to move your limbs in their full range of motion. With *Four Way Burn*, you'll improve your strength in a functional way. You lift a light weight while moving your body in many directions. Your strength gains accumulate naturally and proportionally around your body. Your flexibility improves at the same rate. You can apply your physical improvements to real-world uses.

Working your body parts over and over in isolation, doing the same movements, also creates another problem: Your mind doesn't have to stay involved in your activity. You "zone out" and think about how much longer you must exercise, or you look at the television or listen to the radio in the workout room. You miss out on an opportunity to train your mind to feel and control your body parts while they're in motion, which helps you to prevent injuries.

I believe in the 100 percent approach. Each workout needs to utilize 100 percent of your body and your mind. When you watch TV, listen to music, or daydream while working out, I can guarantee you that part of your focus is going into the program, and part is going into the pounding beat and the singing. If you're not giving 100 percent, you're not going to get 100 percent of the benefit.

Your mind needs to stay active as you move. Your brain picks up signals from your feet and hands and sends messages back to keep you properly balanced. Your brain needs to stay focused on making sure you're maintaining good form.

The fitness industry has created the myth that we need machines and many different exercise tools to stay well, healthy, and fit. Please don't believe it. Your mind and your body are the ultimate training devices, and this program will help you develop them fully.

Weight machines and heavy lifting aren't the only popular forms of exercise that don't allow your body to develop fully. Let's look at a few others to help learn how these differ from the *Four Way Burn* approach. I am *not* discrediting these types of exercise or tools, since many do yield some benefits. But none does a good job of integrating all the aspects of fitness.

Yoga. The emphasis in yoga is on extreme stretching and, in most methods of yoga, holding positions, which can yield *some* benefits. But frankly, there's a lot more to moving than holding yourself in static positions. We normally don't sit around in poses. Doing so overburdens some areas of your body and neglects others, which can cause injuries.

Changing spontaneously in different directions is the way the body performs best. However, "multitasking," such as doing different things with different body parts at the same time, is not taught in yoga. And that's what utilizes the core muscles the most.

Additionally, the cardiovascular (aerobic and anaerobic) system generally is not utilized in yoga. We need both energy systems for activities. In yoga you will not burn many calories.

Medicine balls. When you go to a gym you'll see medicine balls lying around with very few people actually using them. Most of these balls are too heavy, too large, too hard, and too intimidating. You might think a rubber ball that's "only" 8 or 9 pounds isn't very heavy, until you start having to move with it. Your mind wonders, "What do you want me to do with that thing?"

You need strong arms, hands, core muscles, and upper and lower body muscles to throw a heavy medicine ball. If your body parts don't communicate well and you have a poor awareness of how to control your body while in motion, you're likely to get hurt.

But heavy medicine balls *do* make good doorstops.

Pilates. Pilates is not a bad way to get a workout. You strengthen and lengthen your muscles and you work on improving your body's symmetry, which are all goals of my program. On the other hand, it doesn't emphasize free movement. Some Pilates exercises require equipment and some require you to sit, which limits your movements and doesn't work your whole body. Pilates practice is also limited in that it doesn't emphasize change of directions, quickness, reaction time, or agility.

In contrast to these options, the program I've devised over the past decade and used with hundreds of clients works your whole body in a functional way. No muscle is ignored, and

Joel Wilkenfeld

As president of Next Model Management, a modeling agency, Joel Wilkenfeld spends a lot of time around people who are in good physical shape. He wants to make sure he looks and feels his best, too—and some other workouts he's tried just didn't do the job.

"I used to be more into lifting weights, which bulked me up but didn't make me feel better. I've been working with Ralf about 2 years now, and it's more fun than any exercise I've ever done," he says. "It definitely gives me more energy. It makes me feel 100 percent better when I do it."

The 46-year-old still has plenty of strength now, but it's balanced with flexibility—which is one of the central improvements that people will achieve with the *Four Way Burn* program.

"I'd recommend everyone try it and give it some time," Joel urges. "Sometimes it looks easy, but when you do the workouts consistently, there's nothing easy about it."

each body part is encouraged to work with the others. You move as you do in the real world—not just in straight lines.

The *Four Way Burn* program uses 40 techniques—some of which are simple movements, and some of which require more complex motions—to strengthen your entire body and improve your flexibility. As you progress through the techniques, your mind must be an active participant. You're moving in many directions and constantly challenging your balance and coordination. By conditioning your mind and body parts at the same time, you'll allow your nervous system and muscles to perform better in an active lifestyle.

Carol Browne

Carol's home was always filled with active kids. Her oldest son once traveled on an adventure to the Andes Mountains in South America. The next son played high school football. Her third son played lacrosse, and her youngest son plays squash. I've spent time with all of her sons to improve their stamina, flexibility, and strength on the playing field (or the mountain range) of their choice. I've worked with Carol for 14 years and with her husband, too.

"I had worked with someone else for quite a while, and we basically did the same workout over and over. That's typical with a lot of trainers. But Ralf is motivating and challenging, and he mixes things up so it's different," says Carol, who's 57.

"Ralf never believes in exercising one body part at a time. He really makes you feel like you're getting ready for doing something in real life. For a long time, Ralf has been concerned about core body strength, which makes you stronger, with less risk of injury from sports," she says.

2

FOUR WAY BURN WILL CHANGE YOUR LIFE

When you see kids playing, they're often throwing or kicking a ball back and forth to each other. Perhaps it's a baseball, or a football, or a soccer ball. Many times it also takes some sort of ball to lure adults into physical activity, such as a tennis ball or golf ball. That's because playing with a ball is naturally fun.

Exercising just for the sake of exercising, however, can quickly become boring or tedious, especially if you're not really mentally engaged. The more you exercise and the longer you do it, the more likely you'll try to find an excuse to get out of it.

Even losing weight is not enough of an incentive. You either lose weight, at which point you feel less need to exercise, or you become so tired of "having to" exercise that it becomes a chore like vacuuming. Since you only get out of your workouts what you put into them, as soon as you stop moving your body, you stop reaping the benefits.

But becoming fit and healthy takes time, just as it takes former smokers time to clear the effects of cigarette smoke from their bodies. Your fitness program should be slow, progressive, and enjoyable enough to keep you doing it for the long term. You need to strengthen your entire musculoskeletal system and make it flexible so that you can move properly again. And you should stick with the program long enough to ensure that your new habits become ingrained and you can maintain them with little effort.

That's why my program involves a ball.

Working with a ball will keep you engaged. You will focus on using your body to move the ball through the space around you. It's a challenge to control the ball and make it travel where you want it to go. Your exercise now has a purpose besides burning a certain number of calories or sweating for half an hour. If you were to go out into an empty field and run as fast as you could while switching directions and kicking and diving at random, it wouldn't be much fun. But when you add a soccer ball to your activity, it has a purpose. It's fun.

This program is an invitation to you to move again. I want you to feel the sense of playfulness again that you had as a child. With this program, you'll learn 40 activities that require you to engage in both simple and complex motions while controlling a ball.

While holding the ball, you'll extend your arms, bend down and stand up, and twist and turn. You'll soon be able to pass the ball through your legs and around your body. Everyone who's reasonably healthy can do these techniques, from beginners to advanced athletes. All this pushing, pulling, twisting, and turning improves your balance and coordination, agility, quickness, reaction time, and footwork. You'll also increase your joint stability, which protects your joints from injury.

While you're at it, you'll build skills that your body is lacking. If you're strong but not flexible and coordinated (which is the case for many men), you'll enhance your flexibility. If you're very limber but not strong (the case for many women), you'll improve your strength.

And this is a program you can stick with for a long time. Karate students practice groups of motions called *kata*, which are a series of very precise kicks, strikes, and blocks. You'd think it would be easy to master a kata. But martial arts practitioners practice them over and over for years on end—often for their entire lives. These activities keep teaching them new things about how to control their bodies as they move through different positions.

The techniques in the *Four Way Burn* program aren't about karate or self-defense, but they do offer you the same benefits for improving your mobility.

Here's how it works: Each month for 4 months, you'll work through a new cycle of 10 techniques. The groups of movements start simple and grow more complex. I want these activities to be motions that you'll enjoy practicing for year after year—not just for a few months until you lose weight or an injury subsides. Once you feel how much your function improves, you'll want to stick with it.

I've designed the program so that you can keep making the moves a little more complicated to add to the challenge. These activities should become more challenging as you grow more fit—they should never feel stale.

If you regularly run or bicycle, or play tennis or golf, I've created special versions of the program just for you. For most of the year, you can do the regular *Four Way Burn* program, then you can shift to the specialized program before you start playing the sport frequently (such as during the summer) to get ready for it.

THE SPECIAL BENEFITS OF THE PROGRAM

One of the best qualities of this program is that it provides many kinds of improvements to your fitness in one short workout session. You don't have to devote 30 minutes to lifting weights, another 30 minutes to aerobic exercise, and more time to warmup and cooldown sessions before and after exercise.

Emme

When supermodel and television host Emme spends time conditioning her body, she wants to feel the results from her core muscles all the way out to her fingertips. That's why she's a big fan of doing *Four Way Burn* techniques.

"When Ralf and I work with each other, I always walk away and say, 'Oh my God, this is the most thorough workout I've ever done.' I really think of it as the 'full body, even your fingertips are sore' workout," she says. "I've never been so fully trained in every muscle everywhere!"

A former college rower who describes herself as a "high-level athlete," Emme puts a lot of emphasis on conditioning the core muscles of her abdomen and back and the other muscle groups that tie into them.

"If you don't have that core tight and strong, you won't be strong everywhere else. It's like the foundation of your home. If the foundation has leaks in the basement, the rest of the structure of the house will be weak," she says.

As a plus-size model, Emme has made a priority of raising awareness through her public appearances and books that fitness doesn't just mean "skinny."

"My goal is to encourage fitness for all ages and sizes, and it's ridiculous to think you have to be ultra-thin to be considered fit. I know people who are more rounded who are triathletes and they train every day. Compare them with someone who is very trim and considered to be 'fit,' but who doesn't work out. The person who's more full-figured and more athletic is truly the more fit and healthy person," she says.

Because you get four main benefits from each workout, I decided to call the program *Four Way Burn*. Here's a closer look at each of the four ways that every single workout will improve your body.

Benefit #1: Total mind and body conditioning. Too many other types of exercise don't require much mental involvement. While running on a treadmill, you can watch TV. While lifting weights, you may simply focus on counting your number of repetitions.

With *Four Way Burn*, you do complex movements that require careful mental focus to make sure you're holding your body in good form and breathing properly. In addition, you work all parts of your body equally. We tend to focus our workouts on the tasks that are easiest or that we enjoy doing the most. We end up ignoring some of our body parts. You probably have better coordination and strength in your dominant hand (the right hand, for most of us). If so, you're probably weaker on your left side.

Four Way Burn requires you to use both sides of your body equally well. Your muscles and brain grow accustomed to this new challenge, which enables you to control your body better.

Benefit #2: Cardiovascular and pulmonary fitness. While doing these activities, you'll breathe regularly and deeply, in and out, in and out. You don't hold your breath, as you may be tempted to do while lifting weights. Without proper breathing technique, the central nervous system quickly sends messages to your body to preserve the remaining oxygen. Your muscles suffer, causing you to grow tense and tight.

Deep breathing will allow both your vital organs and your muscles to keep working. It will keep your mind sharp and focused on each task at hand. And since deep breathing uses your diaphragm and the deep layers of your abdominal muscles, these areas get more of a workout.

You also won't stop between each activity, or you'll stop only for a moment or two if necessary. This keeps your heart rate and respiration elevated, giving your heart and lungs a good workout and improving their capacity.

Benefit #3: Lengthening and strengthening and joint stability. Too many forms of exercise cause your muscles to grow heavy and tight, pulling your body out of its proper balance. With *Four Way Burn*, you use a small weight—only 4 to 6 pounds—and you constantly stretch out your body. You stand up tall and fully extend your arms and legs. As a result, your muscles become the *opposite* of bulky and restrained. I'm constantly telling my clients to "think long and strong" as they work with the ball, and that lengthening and strengthening are what this workout will do for you.

In addition, your feet, knees, hips, shoulders, and elbows are surrounded by small muscles that keep the joints stabilized. Most of the time when you work out, you don't really give these small muscles a chance to perform. Instead, your bigger muscles—your biceps, your pectorals, your quadriceps—pick up the load.

The small stabilizing muscles only get to perform when your arms and legs are fully extended. As a result, many of these 40 activities require you to bring your arms and legs out straight. They're not "locked" or hyperextended, but they're nearly as straight as you can make them. And since the weight you're maneuvering isn't heavy, bigger muscles don't step in and take up the load. The little muscles around your joints grow stronger, holding each joint in its proper position.

Another benefit to moving your joints through their full range of motion is decreased wear and tear. According to my colleague Evan Karas, MD, "Range of motion distributes force across the entire joint. For instance, if you're having a little bit of arthritis in your knee and you're trying to exercise and take some of the pressure off your knee, if you're not moving your joint through a full range of motion, there will be much more wear in one location of the joint, rather than distributing the force throughout the entire joint, so it would wear more slowly."

This program is also particularly good for stabilizing the feet. Your feet play a crucial role in providing signals to your brain so that it can track and control your body's positioning as you move. But most people's feet are not especially strong, and their feet can't provide this information. Weak feet lead to imbalances in the knees, hips, and spine. During the *Four Way Burn* program, your feet grow strong and are better able to keep your body in good balance.

Benefit #4: Increased calorie burn now and later. Most forms of aerobic exercise use only your legs, not your upper body (although cross-country skiing and rowing are two exceptions). That means a lot of your muscles are burning few calories during your workout. *Four Way Burn* brings all your muscles into the action: your arms, chest, back, abdomen, buttocks, and legs. All of your muscles will burn calories, making this program a much better choice for weight loss than many others.

In addition, the *Four Way Burn* workout increases your metabolism, which means you'll burn calories at a higher level for several hours after each session.

Those are the big four improvements you'll get from sticking with this program, but there are many other benefits, too.

- You'll work your core muscles from many different directions. Situps and crunches require very simple, lateral movements that don't prepare your body for how it really moves. With *Four Way Burn*, you move a weighted ball above your core and work your hips and legs below, so your core must control and transfer energy from both directions.
- Your arms and legs will learn to work better together. You'll also improve your reaction time, agility, and power. These are all skills that will improve your performance in many sports and that will also help you in your everyday life—whether you're walking down busy sidewalks or maneuvering through a crowded toy store during the holidays.
- You'll improve your sense of well-being as your body and mind grow more connected.

Nancy Simpkins

More than 30 years ago, Nancy's cousin went on an Outward Bound adventure, a program that challenges participants to test their physical limits in an outdoor setting.

As the years went by, Nancy kept thinking about her cousin's trip, wondering whether she would have the endurance to finish the program, too. "Wouldn't it be wonderful to accomplish this and feel the way my cousin did?" she would ask herself. In her late forties, she finally decided to quit thinking about it and actually sign up for the trip.

"I knew I'd be carrying a 45-pound pack, and it was going to require some specific training. I was active, but I didn't have any sort of regular exercise program," she says.

Nancy had been participating for several years in a group class that I led, and she began working with me on an individual basis to improve the specific skills she'd need for her adventure. She gradually strengthened her arms and legs, improved her stamina and balance, and departed for Colorado prepared for white-water rafting, rock climbing, and hiking up a 14,000-foot mountain.

Nancy, the mother of two grown children, still works with me regularly to maintain her fitness so she can keep meeting the challenges of her active lifestyle.

"I'm probably more fit at 50 than I was at 25," she says. "I'm a tennis player and a skier and with both of those activities, you're often moving in more than one direction at once— you're turning, bending, and reaching. And Ralf is very good at creating exercises that are functional for my particular lifestyle.

"We also do a lot of exercises that incorporate balance," she says. "Your sense of balance is so key to anything you're doing, from standing to running to any other exercise. If your stance is balanced when you're hitting a tennis ball, you're going to hit the ball better. It minimizes your fatigue and maximizes technique."

Exercise also makes your body produce endorphins, natural chemicals that make you feel relaxed and refreshed.

▶ You'll become even more fit as you follow the principle of *cycling*. You'll gradually put new challenges and demands on your body, and once it can perform at a new level, you'll increase the challenge a little more. Since you'll slowly increase your performance, the higher level of wellness and fitness willl become your new norm. Additionally, with the concept of consistent progression, you will have a low risk of injury.

GETTING STARTED

As I mentioned earlier, the *Four Way Burn* program involves four 1-month cycles, each of which contains 10 techniques. The movements that you'll do during the first month are relatively simple. You'll get the hang of maintaining the proper form and moving your body smoothly, without having to master any particularly complicated moves. At the end of the month, you'll be prepared to handle the new levels of challenge that follow.

All you need for this program is a ball and a little bit of floor space. I have my clients work out with a ball that I designed specially for this program, called the Performance Ball. It's the size of a small beach ball and filled with a dense, rigid foam. The ball, available in 4- and 6-pound options, can be purchased at www.performanceball.com.

Its large size puts your shoulders in the proper position when you hold the ball in front of your chest with both hands. It's soft, allowing you to dig your fingers into it so you get a good finger and hand workout. Plus, it won't hurt if you drop it on your toes. Its shell is made of a fabric that doesn't get slippery if your hands become sweaty.

Though this program was designed with the Performance Ball in mind, you can use one of the following options instead.

▶ **A light medicine ball.** I know I voiced my displeasure with heavy medicine balls in the last chapter, but using a light medicine ball—4 or 6 pounds—is a reasonable choice for this program. Just don't exceed 6 pounds. You'll have trouble controlling a heavy ball through these complex movements, and it will slow down your natural pace and throw off your balance. Try to find a medicine ball with a large diameter—at least as big as a basketball—if possible.

▶ **A beach ball and wrist weights.** An inexpensive way to work out with the proper weight *and* a ball big enough to hold your shoulders in the proper position is to use an inflatable beach ball while wearing light weights strapped to your wrists. These weights are similar to the weighted cuffs that you wear on your ankles, but they are made specifically for your wrists. Get a pair that weighs 2 to 3 pounds each, and make sure they fit snugly, but not too tightly, on your wrists.

Difficulty level

Each of these techniques has three levels of difficulty: beginner, intermediate, and advanced. This way you can continue with the program over the long term without becoming bored, even as you grow more skilled and comfortable with the movements. I'd recommend that most people start at the beginner or intermediate level. However, the questionnaire on page 28 can tell you your ideal starting point. In general, once you pick a difficulty level, stick with it until you've completed your four cycles. However, you're certainly free to play with different elements to make a technique a little harder if you need more of a challenge. You'll see the directions on how to bump up the difficulty level before each technique's description.

Moving through each session's format

During each session, you will perform techniques 1 through 3, then repeat them a second time. You then move through 4 through 7, then run through them again. You then move through 8 through 10, then repeat them for a second set.

This means you'll do *two* sets of each activity. The first set will establish communication between your mind and your body and get them working in unison. The second set is to reinforce your skills and your muscle memory and build stamina. You'll also burn calories and strengthen your muscles with each set.

As you progress through the weeks in each cycle, you'll be doing more repetitions of each exercise during each set. You'll find a chart at the end of each chapter that summarizes the number of reps and sets you should do for each technique.

Timing of your sessions

You'll get the maximum benefit from *Four Way Burn* by performing three sessions a week. I recommend that you space these out so that you're not doing them on back-to-back days.

On your "off" days, do a different form of sport, a group aerobics program, or some other physical activity that you enjoy.

However, if you're extremely active or you're training for a big event and need to practice that sport every day, do your *Four Way Burn* session at the opposite time of day. For example, do *Four Way Burn* in the morning and your other activity in the late afternoon or evening, or vice versa. Make sure that, if you're conditioning yourself day after day, you take one day each week as a rest day to allow your body to recover and recuperate.

No need for warmups or cooldowns

The flexibility training built into each activity means that you don't have to stretch before or after a *Four Way Burn* session. Remember that this is a lengthening and strengthening program, so you will stretch your muscles sufficiently.

Your warmup is embedded in the first three techniques within each program. That's why it's important to follow the techniques in the sequence in which they are described.

Avoid distractions

Find a quiet place without a television, radio, telephone, or other distractions. If you decide to follow this program at the gym, I'd also suggest that you avoid looking at yourself in the mirror during the activity.

It is important that you focus on your body's movements. Feeling your movements allows your sensory system to replace your visual cues. This allows your proprioception—or sense of body movement—to control and lead your body in motion.

In addition, using a mirror slows down your reaction time and takes away valuable attention, which should be used to reinforce your mind-body communication.

As you perform these activities, simply "gaze" out into the room as you focus your mind on your movements.

Go barefoot

You'll get a better feel for the positioning of your feet if you don't wear shoes. Going barefoot improves your overall sense of positioning. If you must wear shoes, use new ones that haven't been broken in doing other sports.

Switch sides

In order to improve your balance and symmetry, when you do any technique that requires you to use a single arm or a single leg, be sure to do the same number of repetitions on the opposite side, unless instructed differently. We have a natural tendency to always start off on the dominant side, which leads to lopsidedness and a lack of balance. By switching off, you give your weaker side more attention, bringing your body into better balance.

Take your time

Don't rush through these movements. In the charts at the end of each chapter, I have suggested a minimum and maximum length of time that each workout should take. By taking plenty of time, you can move at a deliberate pace so that each joint moves through its entire range of motion. This works each joint at its weakest angle, thus strengthening its stabilizing muscles.

During the first 6 to 8 weeks of the program, your body will have to relearn how it moves. Your many parts will become accustomed to communicating with each other and working together better. Your body took many years to develop its current habits, and it'll take a while for it to get used to a new way of moving. Just stick with it. The following weeks and months will really build up your strength, flexibility, and heart and lung functioning.

PART

PROGRESSIVE CYCLES MOVE YOU TO SUCCESS

3

THE FIRST CYCLE

Are you ready? It's time to start learning how to do the techniques. Just remember to breathe regularly and in rhythm with each exercise. As long as you remain in control of your body's movements, you can push yourself further than you're accustomed. Stay focused while you perform each task, and enjoy the experience.

As you work through the techniques, make sure you get all the benefits from the program by paying attention to the following factors.

Just get started. You don't need to warm up before a session or stretch afterward. You'll have plenty of stretching during each workout.

Keep your shoulders back and down. Pull your shoulder blades together and hold your upper body up straight and tall. You want to avoid hunching over. This ensures that your rear shoulder girdle becomes strengthened, which helps to improve your posture.

"Suck and tuck." This is my way of telling clients how to keep their pelvis in the right position. Your pelvis should be tilted forward. This requires you to tighten your abdominal muscles and pull your buttocks in. The opposite—and incorrect—posture would be to have your buttocks pushed out, your belly jutting out, and your lower back in a "swayback" position.

Keep a narrow stance. For most of these 40 movements, your feet should be at shoulder width or narrower. You might be tempted to widen your stance to improve your balance. However, when you do this, you settle into a position that doesn't require you to work as hard to maintain your balance. We want to *challenge* your body—not make things easier for it.

Keep a strong grip. If you merely let the ball rest in your hands, you miss a lot of the benefits of this workout. Really dig your fingers and hands into the ball throughout the entire

(continued on page 30)

What's Your Proper Starting Level?

Check with your doctor before beginning this or any exercise program. Ask yourself the following questions to determine at which difficulty level to start the program.

If you can answer yes to any of these questions, discuss the issues with your doctor:

▶ Do you experience shortness of breath even when you're not moving?

▶ Do you have unexplained fatigue, weakness, or dizziness?

▶ Do you have flulike symptoms, such as sweating or nausea?

▶ Do you smoke or have high blood pressure or high cholesterol?

▶ Have you had any kind of surgery within the past 3 months?

▶ Have you had any injuries within the past 6 weeks?

▶ Have you recently been prescribed a physical therapy program?

▶ Are you pregnant?

▶ Do you lose your balance when you change directions?

▶ Are you unable to climb stairs?

▶ Are you unable to dress or undress?

▶ Are you unable to lie down on the floor and stand up without help?

▶ Are you unable to maintain the hygiene of your lower extremities?

▶ Are you unable to get in and out of a bathtub without assistance?

▶ Do you wear ankle, knee, back, wrist, or elbow braces?

▶ Are you unable to walk while carrying items?

▶ Are you unable to walk more than 5 minutes without stopping?

▶ Are you unable to move from a sitting to a standing position?

▶ Do you perceive your health as poor?

Start at the beginner level if you answer yes to all or most of these questions:

▶ Have you completed a physical therapy program within the past 2 weeks?

▶ Are you still in pain after trying all the modern methods of pain management?

▶ Can you make your bed, including changing the sheets and pillows?

▶ Do you do light housework, like dusting, washing dishes, and mopping?

▶ Do you prepare your own meals?

▶ Do you shop for your own groceries?

▶ Do you periodically experience neck and shoulder stiffness?

▶ Do you feel sleepless at night?

▶ Do you experience stiffness in any joints?

▶ Do you have difficulty getting in and out of the shower?

▶ Do you exercise less than 30 minutes, 3 days per week?

▶ Are you unable to squat without lifting your heels off the floor?

- Are you unable to interlock your fingers behind your head?
- Can you stand on each foot for up to 30 seconds?
- Can you pick up an object from a location over your head?

- If you play golf, do you use a cart?
- Are you often tired during the day?
- Do you exercise on an inflatable ball?
- Do you perceive your health as fair?
- Can you exercise 15 to 20 minutes at a low to moderate pace?

Start at the intermediate level if you answer yes to all or most of these questions:

- Do you garden regularly?
- Can you stand on each foot for at least 1 minute?
- Can you lift objects that weigh 5 to 6 pounds from the table, chair, or floor?
- If you play golf, do you walk?
- Do you have a job that requires frequent driving?
- Do you lift heavy weights?
- Do you practice yoga or Pilates?
- Do you regularly use free weights or rubber bands for exercise?
- Can you walk nonstop for a mile or two?

- Can you walk slow and fast, backward, and with changing directions?
- Do you jog or run on different types of surfaces?
- Can you swim with an overhead stroke and backstroke?
- Can you move different-sized objects at different speeds?
- Do you exercise at least two times per week?
- Do you perceive your health as good?
- Can you exercise 15 to 20 minutes three times per week?

Start at the advanced level if you answer yes to all or most of these questions:

- Can you run in circles, figure eights, and side shuffles?
- Can you jump vertically, forward, sideways, and backward?
- Can you throw various objects under-hand, overhand, or with two hands?
- Can you catch different-sized and -weighted balls with one or two hands?
- Can you hit a baseball with a bat or a tennis ball with a racket?

- Do you play active court sports at least 2 days a week?
- Do you exercise four or more times per week?
- Do you practice any form of martial art?
- Are you an endurance athlete?
- Can you stand on each foot for at least $1\frac{1}{2}$ minutes?
- Do you perceive your health as excellent?

range of motion. You'll increase the strength of your fingers, hands, wrists, forearms, upper arms, and chest.

You'll be able to open cans and bottles more easily, you'll help prevent carpal tunnel syndrome, and you'll perform better in sports that require you to control a racket or throw a ball.

Keep breathing. Never hold your breath during these techniques. You need to breathe in and out regularly. For each technique, I'll recommend moments when you should blow your breath out.

Richard Handler

As CEO of a global banking and securities firm, Richard has a stressful, physically challenging job that demands a lot of focus and stamina.

So when he has time in his busy schedule for a workout, he doesn't want to waste it "just getting bigger arms and a bigger neck." He wants one workout that improves *all* the aspects of his fitness at one time.

That's why Richard, the CEO of Jefferies Group, Inc., has been working with me regularly for nearly 6 years. "How I feel is very important. If I feel like I'm in good shape and I have my workouts in a good routine, I'm just in a good place physically and I'm a better person intellectually."

Before working with the *Four Way Burn* techniques, Richard knew he had "bad posture and terrible flexibility, and lingering lower back and neck pains from playing sports growing up," he says.

Now his posture is better, and so are his flexibility and upper body strength. His chronic pains still flare up "a little, but nowhere near what they used to be."

And with four kids and a hectic life, the 44-year-old needs to squeeze a lot of conditioning out of the brief periods he can allot to physical activity. "When you're done working out with Ralf, you know you've worked out!" he adds.

Push and Pull

Beginner: Follow the directions below.

Intermediate: Stand in a split stance: knees bent and feet flat on the floor about shoulder-width apart, with one foot placed in front of the other.

Advanced: Start in a split stance, with your back foot up on the ball of the foot.

Emphasizes: Rear shoulder girdle, chest, arms, triceps, and core muscles (these aren't just your abs and lower back, but also the connecting muscles in your torso and between your arms and chest).

Functional improvements: Better posture and body alignment, proprioception (mind and body connection), and kinesthetic awareness; improved symmetry (balance on both sides of your body); preventive rehabilitation for rounded, hunched shoulders; and better awareness of the proper positioning of your upper back.

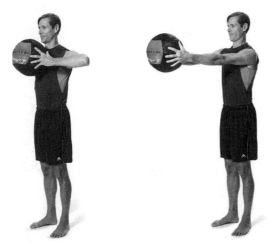

Begin in a parallel stance, which means your feet are side by side and spaced shoulder-width apart. Start by holding the ball at your chest, with your elbows pointed out to the sides. Push the ball out until your arms are fully extended in a "soft lock." Draw the ball back to your chest, and repeat. Breathe out as you push the ball away from you, then inhale, and breathe out again as you pull the ball toward you.

On the first one-third of the repetitions, push the ball straight out. On the next third of the repetitions, push it out diagonally to your left. On the final third of the repetitions, push it out diagonally to your right. While pushing out at an angle, twist your upper body toward that particular side.

DO:

▶ Grip the ball firmly. Really dig your fingertips and palms into it.

▶ Remember to "suck and tuck" your pelvis on this and all the other techniques.

▶ After each repetition, pull the ball back to your chest, firmly pressing it into your sternum.

▶ Squeeze your shoulder blades together and keep your shoulders pressed down.

DON'T:

▶ Slouch or arch your back.

▶ Tilt your head forward or backward.

Saturn

Beginner: Follow the directions below.

Intermediate: Stand in a "crossover" stance, in which you cross one leg over the other, so that your feet are side by side but on opposite sides of each other. Reverse your leg position before beginning the second set.

Advanced: Stand on one leg for the first set, switching legs for the second set.

Emphasizes: Shoulder girdle, rotator cuffs, upper and middle trapezius muscles between your neck and shoulders; your chest, arms, biceps, wrists, and core muscles.

Functional improvements: Prevents rounded shoulders; improves posture; reduces neck discomfort; helps prevent rotator cuff injuries and carpal tunnel syndrome; improves symmetry; improves bloodflow to the central nervous system; and invigorates the body.

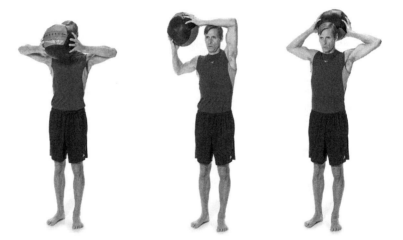

Stand in a parallel stance with your feet less than shoulder-width apart. Grip the ball in both hands in front of your face, with your elbows pointed outward. Now rotate the ball around your head in a circle. As it travels around your head, keep your elbows pointed outward. Breathe out for half of the circle around your head, and breathe in for the other half. When the ball reaches the front of your face, you've completed one repetition.

Do the recommended number of repetitions, then switch directions and repeat for the same number.

DO:

▶ Keep the ball at face level, particularly when you are reaching around the back of your head.

▶ Keep your head motionless and your gaze forward.

▶ Keep your back straight.

▶ Squeeze the ball tightly.

DON'T:

▶ Move your head around.

▶ Touch your head with the ball.

Progressive Cycles Move You to Success

Side Twist

Beginner: Follow the directions below.

Intermediate: Do this in a split stance, with your rear foot resting on the ball of the foot.

Advanced: Follow the intermediate directions, but extend your arms outward. As you reach your maximum motion on each side, look over your shoulder. When you turn to the left, look over your left shoulder, and when you turn to the right, look over your right shoulder.

Emphasizes: Upper body, core muscles, shoulders, neck, lats, waist, and lower back.

Functional improvements: Better spatial awareness and improved equilibrium; improved hip, knee, and ankle stability; better functional and athletic performance.

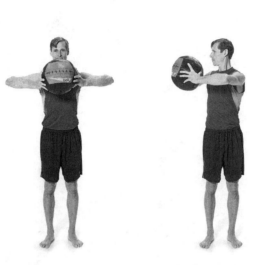

Begin with your feet in a parallel stance, with your hands holding the ball close in front of your chest and your elbows pointing out to the sides. Twist your torso to the side, using the core muscles around your abdomen and lower back to provide movement. Twist only your upper body—do not twist at the knees. Each repetition requires you to fully twist one way, then the other.

Exhale one long breath as you move in each direction.

DO:

▶ Keep your legs motionless—the movement should involve only your core and your torso.

▶ Keep your shoulders relaxed.

▶ Move steadily and smoothly back and forth.

▶ Keep the ball and your elbows at chest height.

DON'T:

▶ Shrug your shoulders upward.

▶ Pivot your knees or move your feet.

▶ Swing your arms. Your movement should come from your trunk.

Rocking Chair

Beginner: Lift the ball as high as you can. If you can only bring it parallel to the floor, that's fine.

Intermediate: Lift the ball at least in the direction of the ceiling.

Advanced: Lift the ball overhead.

Emphasizes: Ankles, calves, shin muscles, plantar fasciae (the tissue between your heel and toes), buttocks, core muscles, chest, and rear shoulder muscles.

Functional improvements: Improves posture, balance, and shoulder flexibility; strengthens posterior shoulder girdle; makes reaching behind or over the head easier; reduces neck and shoulder stiffness; makes lifting and lowering objects overhead easier; strengthens feet and ankles; prevents shinsplints and Achilles tendon tears; and strengthens abdominals and buttocks to support and protect the lower back.

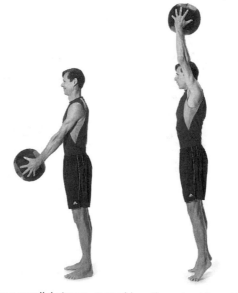

Begin with your feet in a parallel stance, spaced less than shoulder-width apart. Stand up straight and hold the ball so that it's hanging down in front of your groin, with your arms fully extended.

Rise up on your toes as you bring the ball straight overhead. Your arms should remain fully extended—never bending—at all times. Lower the ball back to the starting position as you rock back onto your heels to complete one repetition.

Breathe out as you rock your feet forward, and again as you rock your feet backward.

DO:

▶ Keep your head and back aligned.
▶ Go at a speed at which you can maintain good control.
▶ Come up onto the balls of your feet.

DON'T:

▶ Bend forward.
▶ Move your hips forward and backward.
▶ Raise the ball behind your head—it should stop when it's directly overhead.
▶ Roll on the outsides of your feet.

Squat and Push

Emphasizes: Chest, posterior shoulder girdle, shoulders, lower back, buttocks, legs, core muscles, and feet.

Functional improvements: Prevents lower back, knee, and hip pain, especially after sitting or standing for long periods; improves functional and athletic performance; promotes body symmetry, better posture, and easier movement; and stretches and strengthens the Achilles tendons.

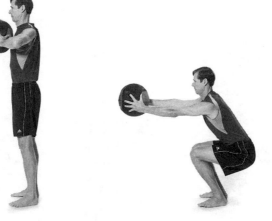

Begin in a parallel stance. Start by holding the ball in front of your chest with your elbows pointed outward. Now squat down. As you squat, fully extend the ball away from you until your arms are straightened in a soft lock. Look straight ahead at all times.

As you squat, keep your feet flat—don't rise up on your toes. As you stand up, simultaneously pull the ball back to your chest and squeeze your shoulder blades together to complete one repetition. Take in one deep breath going down, exhale, and take another deep breath coming up. Work toward squatting more deeply with each repetition.

DO:

▶ Keep your feet flat on the floor.
▶ Keep your knees aligned over your feet.
▶ Keep your back straight.
▶ Stick your tailbone out when squatting down.

DON'T:

▶ Rise up onto your toes as you squat.
▶ Hunch or round your shoulders.

Hula Hoop

Beginner: Keep your eyes open.

Intermediate: Close your eyes.

Advanced: Close your eyes, and take one step out and then back to center as you do this movement. Alternating between feet, step forward as the ball goes behind you, to one side when it goes past the other hip, then back as it passes in front of you, and so forth.

Emphasizes: The lateral muscles at the side of your back; the core muscles, shoulders, upper and lower back, hips, arms, wrists, hands, and fingers.

Functional improvements: Improves grip strength; relieves joint soreness in hands and fingers; reduces stiffness and tightness of neck, lower back, and hips; loosens tight chest and shoulder muscles; improves reaction time, body symmetry, proprioception, and kinesthetic awareness (awareness of body position, weight, or movement of the body); and improves coordination between different body parts.

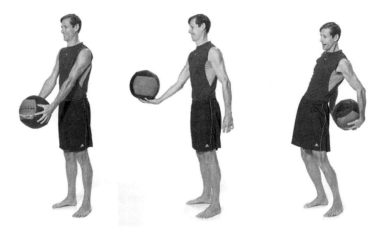

Begin with your feet parallel and close together. Grip the ball firmly between both hands and hold it in front of your abdomen. Start rotating the ball around your body, scooping it up from hand to hand as it passes your midsection and back. Much like a hula hoop, it should travel smoothly around and around your body.

Rotate your hips as the ball passes around your body. Breathe out as the ball passes behind your back and again when it goes across your front. Complete all your repetitions in one direction, then repeat in the other direction.

DO:

▶ Scoop the ball up behind your back.
▶ Move at a speed that allows you to stay in control of the ball.

DON'T:

▶ Roll the ball against your body—keep it controlled in your hands.
▶ Try to throw from hand to hand.

Progressive Cycles Move You to Success

Thigh Kick and Catch

Beginner: After each repetition, touch your foot firmly back to the floor.

Intermediate: After each repetition, only allow your foot to lightly touch the floor.

Advanced: After each repetition, do not lower your foot all the way back to the floor.

Emphasizes: Thighs, hip flexors, buttocks, ankle stabilizers, core muscles, chest, shoulders.

Functional improvements: Strengthens ankles and hips; improves balance and coordination; improves focus, proprioception, and kinesthetic awareness; and allows faster response time to situations at work, traveling, or at play.

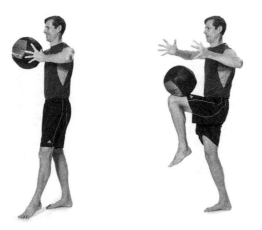

Start with most of your weight on one foot and the other foot lightly touching the floor in front of you. Grip the ball in front of your chest with your elbows pointed outward. Lift your knee straight up in front of you and drop the ball so that it bounces off of your upper thigh. The ball should only bounce up a few inches. At the height of its bounce, grab the ball and lower your leg to the starting position to complete one repetition. Exhale with each kick. Complete all the repetitions with one foot, then repeat with the other foot.

DO:

▶ Maintain good control over the ball. If you're losing control, slow down.

DON'T:

▶ Hit the ball so hard with your thigh that it bounces more than a few inches.

▶ Push the ball down to your leg. Instead, drop it.

Soldier Walk

Beginner: Repeat with the same leg until you finish the set, then switch to the other leg.

Intermediate: Switch legs with each repetition.

Advanced: Use the same leg until you finish your set, but don't lower your foot all the way to the floor between repetitions.

Emphasizes: Thighs, hamstrings, buttocks, chest, core muscles, shoulders, and arms.

Functional improvements: Improved balance and coordination; more dynamic flexibility in the lower back, hips, and hamstrings; and a stronger grip.

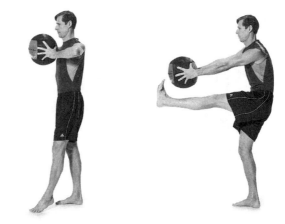

Begin with most of your weight on one foot and the other lightly touching the floor in front of you. Grip the ball in front of your chest with elbows pointed outward. Lift your front leg up while keeping it extended. At the same time, push the ball straight out, exhale, and touch it to your lower shin when your leg reaches its maximum height. Keeping your leg straight, lower your foot back to the floor and pull the ball back to your chest to complete one repetition.

DO:

► Lean over from your hips.
► Lift your leg at a constant speed rather than in a jerking motion.

DON'T:

► Bend the knee of the swinging leg.
► Hunch over.

Progressive Cycles Move You to Success

Good Morning

Beginner: Try to touch the ball to the floor farther away from your feet.

Intermediate: Do this technique from a split stance, in which you take a half-step forward with one foot, rather than using a parallel stance.

Advanced: Reach out as far from your body as you can with the ball, then drop it and catch it after it bounces off the floor.

Emphasizes: Hamstrings, lower back, calves, and core muscles.

Functional improvements: Improves symmetry and alignment; prevents injuries to lower back, hips, hamstrings, and calves; allows you to sit or stand longer without stiffness; and strengthens the muscles on your backside that are needed to counterbalance muscles in the front.

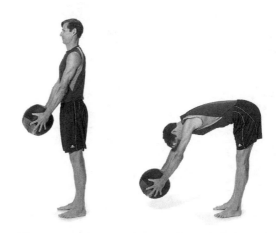

Begin with your feet parallel and less than shoulder-width apart. Bend over at your hips and hold the ball with your arms fully extended downward. Push the ball down to the floor near your feet, or as close to the floor as you can. Put most of your weight on the balls of your feet, but don't lift your heels from the floor.

Stand most of the way back up, but not completely upright, while keeping your arms fully extended toward the floor to complete the repetition. Exhale as you move in each direction.

DO:

► Bend over so you feel the stretch in your lower back.
► Stick your buttocks out.
► Keep your legs straight.
► Create an even arch in your spine as you bend, lifting your tailbone up.

DON'T:

► Bend over using your upper back.
► Hunch or slouch.

Discus

Beginner: Follow the directions below.

Intermediate: Stand in a crossover stance, with your legs crossed and your feet on opposite sides of each other.

Advanced: Stand only on the leg opposite from the hand that's holding the ball. When you switch hands, switch legs.

Emphasizes: Chest, arms, elbows, shoulders, and core muscles.

Functional improvements: Improves flexibility in chest and shoulders; helps prevent elbow tendinitis and wrist strains and sprains; improves shoulder stability and helps prevent shoulder injuries; improves reach, posture, and awareness of the posterior shoulder girdle.

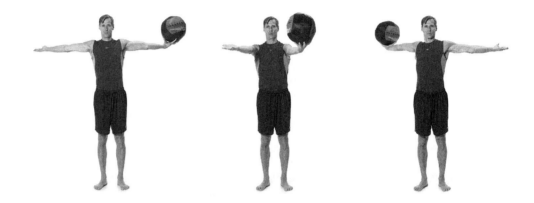

Stand in a parallel stance, with your feet closer than shoulder width apart. Hold the ball in one hand and bring your arm out to your side, keeping your elbow in a soft lock and your arm fully extended the entire time. At the same time, bring your other arm out to your other side, using your full range of motion.

Now bring both hands back in front of you—keeping your arms fully extended—and pass the ball to your empty hand. Bring your arms back out to your sides. Keep repeating and passing the ball from hand to hand. Exhale while reaching out in each direction.

DO:

▶ Grip the ball with your fingertips to control it.
▶ Keep your arms between chest and shoulder height.
▶ Keep your chest and face pointed forward during the entire motion.

DON'T:

▶ Shrug your shoulders.
▶ Lift your arms.
▶ Allow your arms to sag downward.
▶ Twist your torso as you move your arms out to the side.

STRETCHING AND RELAXATION TECHNIQUES

You can rest on your ball to stretch your body as you're taking a break or relaxing after your session is finished. The position I call the Wedge is ideal for use between repetitions. You can also use it after a long day at work or anytime you feel the need to take a load off your back and hips. The Lying Side Twist and the Spread Eagle are ideal after your session is completed. These techniques are also effective after a strenuous day at work or at home, or after an athletic event.

Wedge

Muscle groups primarily relaxed: Shoulders, neck, lower back, buttocks, hamstrings.

Benefits: Instant relief of tight or stiff muscles.

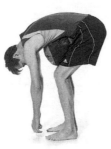

Place the ball between your upper body and your thighs, bend your knees enough to hold the ball in place, and lean over it. Breathe in through your nose and out of your mouth rhythmically. Take just enough time to do this between techniques so that you get your breath back—long enough to take three in-and-out breaths should be enough. When doing this technique after the program, take a little more time with it. Stand up straight, then repeat for a second set if desired.

DO:	DON'T:
▶ Keep your body weight evenly distributed on both feet.	▶ Stop breathing.
▶ Relax your arms and head. Let them hang.	▶ Tense your body. Tension creates tightness.
	▶ Lose your balance.

Lying Side Twist

Muscle groups primarily relaxed: Chest, front shoulder girdle, lower back, buttock, hips, outer thighs, and obliques.

Benefits: Takes the entire body's weight off of the lower back and releases stress and tension in the lower back; also, relaxes your entire body.

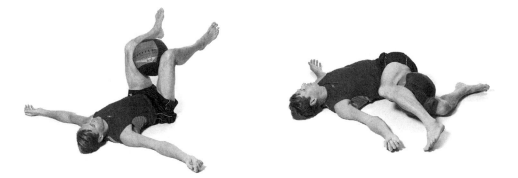

Lie with your back on a firm surface, bend your legs with your feet flat on the floor, and place the ball between your knees and inner thighs. Extend your arms at chest level, your palms facing the ceiling. Press your upper back and head firmly down to the floor.

Now pull your knees toward your chest and lower your legs to the right, rotating at your hips. Your right thigh will end up resting on the floor. Continue to roll your left leg slightly farther over the top of the ball. Now turn your head to the left, and rotate your knees and the ball over to the left.

Breathe deeply in and out of your nose three times while your legs are lowered. Return to the starting position and repeat on your other side. Repeat a second set, if desired.

DO:	DON'T:
▶ Feel the ball firmly between both legs.	▶ Tense up your shoulders, arms, or hands.
▶ Relax your upper body.	▶ Stop breathing.

Spread Eagle

Muscle groups primarily relaxed: Hip flexors and thighs, lower back, knees, and feet.

Benefits: Takes the weight that they carry every day off of your hips and lower back, and creates a better balance in your hips.

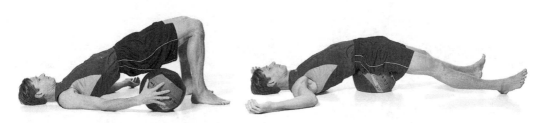

Lie on the floor faceup, with your knees bent and your feet flat on the floor and about hip-distance apart. Lift your hips toward the ceiling so that your body forms a bridge, and wedge the ball under your buttocks. Now spread your arms and legs, as shown. If you have placed the ball too high up under your spine, you will feel a strain in your spine. Reposition the ball so that you feel only a stretch.

Feel your lower back and hips relaxing. Your upper body should be loose. After three breaths in and out of your nose, pull your knees to your chest, keeping the ball wedged between your lower back and the floor. Keep your arms spread out as you pull your knees to your chest, if possible. If you can't bring your knees up without help, use your arms to wrap around your legs for assistance. Hold the stretch for three long breaths, and repeat the cycle.

DO:	DON'T:
▶ Place the ball under your buttocks.	▶ Place the ball under your spine.
▶ Feel the release of tightness around your hips and lower back.	

CYCLE ONE CHART

	WEEK 1 15 to 20 min each program (each daily program includes two sets)	WEEK 2 20 to 25 min each program	WEEK 3 25 to 35 min each program	WEEK 4 35 to 45 min each program
Push and Pull	6 first session 9 second session 12 third session	9 first session 12 second session 15 third session	12 first session 15 second session 18 third session	15 first session 21 second session 27 third session
Saturn, per direction	4 6 8	6 9 10	8 12 15	10 15 20
Side Twist, per direction	5 8 10	7 10 12	10 12 15	12 15 20

Do a second set of the first three techniques, then move to the next group of four.

Rocking Chair	5 8 10	7 10 12	10 12 15	12 15 20
Squat and Push	5 6 10	6 8 12	9 10 15	12 15 20
Hula Hoop, per direction	4 5 8	5 7 10	7 10 15	10 15 20
Thigh Kick and Catch, per leg	6 8 10	8 10 12	10 12 15	10 15 20

Do a second set of the middle four techniques, then move to the last group of three.

Soldier Walk, per leg	5 7 10	7 10 12	9 12 15	12 15 20
Good Morning	5 7 10	7 9 12	10 12 15	12 15 20
Discus, per arm	5 7 10	7 9 12	10 12 15	12 15 20

Do a second set of the final three techniques, then move to the relaxation/stretching techniques below. (See pages 41 to 43.)

Wedge
Lying Side Twist
Spread Eagle

4

THE SECOND CYCLE

After you've worked on basic moves for a month, you'll be ready to progress to a more challenging group of 10 techniques. These techniques will continue to improve your dynamic balance and coordination and your functional strength and flexibility as you move your entire body in a unified way. These new moves will also help create even more coordination between your mind and body.

This program is built on the concept of *cycling*. This means you will progress through cycles that become more and more challenging. When you gradually put more demands on your body, it improves its physical abilities so that it can continue to meet those demands. Your nerves and muscles become better at communicating with each other, and your muscles become stronger.

But your body never becomes overburdened because you don't ask too much of it at any point. That's where injuries such as sprains and strains come from. And taking on a challenge that's too hard too soon can cause you to burn out—and drop out.

The Coil

Emphasizes: Shoulders, arms, hands and fingers, chest, core muscles, midsection, hips, knees and thighs.

Functional improvements: Better coordination, grip strength, body awareness, and symmetry; improves rhythmic and controlled motion, cardiopulmonary efficiency, quickness, and reaction time; and strengthens weak back muscles so they can balance out muscles in the front of the body.

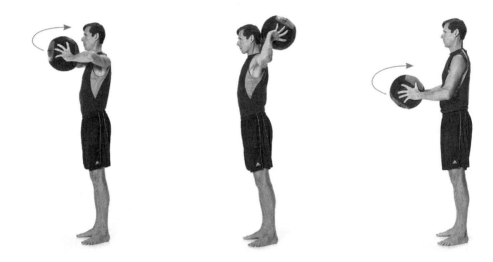

This movement is actually a combination of three techniques, starting with the Saturn (page 32), moving to the Hula Hoop (page 36), and finishing with a new move. To begin, start in the Saturn position. Move the ball around your head, then smoothly lower it and pass it around, behind your midsection. As the ball comes back around to your abdomen, squat down and pass it behind your legs and back in front of you.

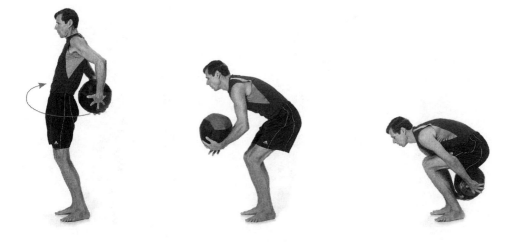

Now, keep moving the ball up and around your body in a Hula Hoop and a Saturn until it ends in front of your face. Going all the way down and all the way up makes one repetition. Exhale as the ball passes in front of you each time.

DO:

▶ Keep your knees together as you squat.

▶ Maintain good control of the ball.

▶ Maintain the good form taught for the Saturn and
  Hula Hoop moves.

Advanced Push and Pull

Beginner: Follow directions below for one set, switching feet for the second set.

Intermediate: Alternate feet with each repetition.

Advanced: With each repetition, jump an inch off the floor while quickly switching your stance. You'll be switching your front and back legs in one sudden motion.

Emphasizes: Chest, shoulders, rear shoulder girdle, core muscles, and legs.

Functional improvements: Better coordination between upper and lower extremities; improves awareness and control of legs and feet while multitasking; better dynamic balance, agility, and footwork; strengthens the knees; and enhances awareness of good posture while moving and carrying objects.

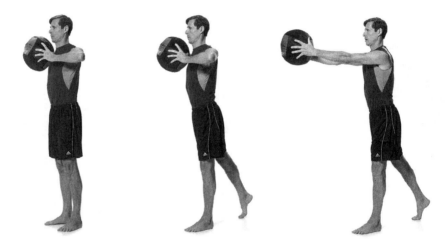

Start with your feet parallel and less than shoulder-width apart. Hold the ball in front of your chest with your elbows pointed outward.

Step forward with one foot while you push the ball out until your arms are straightened in a soft lock. Your back foot should rise up on the ball of the foot.

Bring your front foot back to the starting position as you bring the ball back to your chest to complete the repetition. Exhale with each push and with each pull.

DO:	DON'T:
▶ Keep your arms and the ball at chest height, and keep your body straight.	▶ Drop your elbows and the ball below chest height. ▶ Let your back foot rest flat on the floor.

Diagonal Chop

Beginner: Follow the directions below.

Intermediate: Lift your knee in front of you during the motion of the ball so that you end up standing on one foot. If you chop from the right shoulder to the left hip, lift your left knee up toward your right shoulder. Raise and lower your knee in the opposite direction of the ball's movement, and don't touch the floor with that foot until the repetitions are complete.

Advanced: Start in a deep stance by stepping your right foot forward. Continue by following the intermediate directions. Your left foot will come up off of the floor as the ball goes from your right shoulder to your left hip, and vice versa.

Emphasizes: Chest, shoulders, rotator cuffs, rear shoulder girdle, waist and lower back, buttocks, hips, core muscles, legs, and feet.

Functional improvements: Strengthens rotator cuff support; reduces shoulder stiffness; tightens abdominals; strengthens ankles and feet; improves balance when walking or running; increases smoothness of energy transfer between the arms, shoulder girdle, and lower extremities; and improves muscle strength and muscle memory.

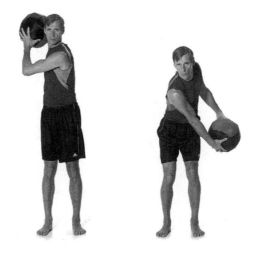

Begin with your feet parallel and less than shoulder-width apart. Hold the ball in both hands over your right shoulder, making sure to not arch your back. Your left shoulder should be relaxed, not shrugged upward, and your torso should be twisted to the right. Maintain a strong grip with both hands.

Move the ball downward toward the floor to your left, taking it on a diagonal path across your body. The ball will end up to the left of your left hip, and your arms will end up straight. Reverse the movement and bring the ball back over your right shoulder to complete the repetition. Complete all repetitions on one side, then switch sides and repeat.

Be sure to breathe out while you're "chopping" the ball down and bringing it up.

DO:

▶ Keep your shoulders relaxed.
▶ "Suck and tuck" your pelvis.
▶ Keep your back straight.

DON'T:

▶ Let your knees touch or cross during the motion.
▶ Hunch over.
▶ Shrug your shoulders upward.
▶ Loosen your grip.

Golfer Swing

Emphasizes: Shoulders, neck, rotator cuffs, core muscles, hips, legs, and feet.

Functional improvements: Improves dynamic balance and kinesthetic awareness; reduces dizziness; improves spatial awareness and peripheral vision; increases confidence and control while changing directions quickly.

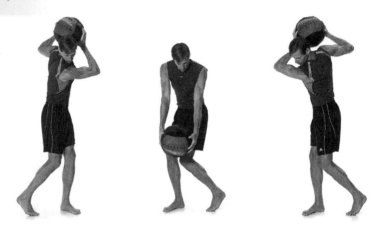

Begin with your feet parallel and close together. Extend your arms and hold the ball in front of your groin.

With both hands, bring the ball up to one shoulder, as if you're setting up to swing a golf club. As you make this motion, pivot the opposite foot (if you turn to your left, it will be your right foot) so it will point toward the direction the ball is traveling. While swinging the ball, only the opposite leg pivots and that foot remains on the ball of the foot. Your entire body will twist as you bring the ball above your shoulder. At the highest point, bend both elbows.

When you reach the highest point, pivot your feet the other way and move the ball back down, across your groin, and up to your other shoulder. Your arms and the ball will look like a pendulum swinging down and up from shoulder to shoulder as your feet pivot back and forth. Inhale when the ball is at its highest point, and exhale forcefully with each swing. Complete all the repetitions on one side, then switch sides and repeat.

DO:

▶ Allow your arms to be fully extended midway through the movement, then bend them to bring the ball to each shoulder.

▶ Pivot your feet and your hips.

▶ Maintain a solid grip.

DON'T:

▶ Loosen your grip.

▶ Jerk your body or wobble.

Statue of Liberty

Beginner: If you can't extend your arm and leg fully, stretch them as far as you can.

Intermediate: Extend your arm and leg more.

Advanced: Extend your arm and leg to the position shown below.

Emphasizes: Neck and shoulders, arms, biceps, rotator cuff, lower back, hips, thighs, core muscles.

Functional improvements: Improves posture, balance, and coordination; strengthens the upper back; protects rotator cuffs from injury; improves throwing and catching skills; improves functional core strength, proprioception, and kinesthetic awareness; increases flexibility while turning your body; improves multitasking ability; and reduces stiffness in the lower back and hips.

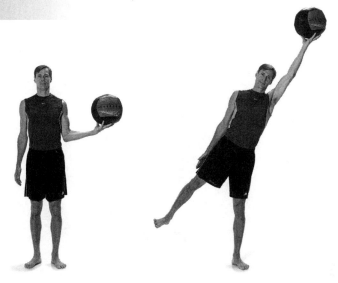

Begin with your feet parallel and just a few inches apart. Hold the ball in one hand, with your arm at your side and bent at a 90-degree angle.

Slowly extend the arm with the ball, reaching up and out over your shoulder as you lift your opposite leg up and out to the side, as shown. Return your arm and your leg to their starting point to complete the repetition. Complete all repetitions on one side, then switch sides and repeat.

Breathe out when your arms and legs come together, and again when they move apart.

DO:	DON'T:
▶ Lift your leg in a controlled manner, not a jerking motion.	▶ Stop breathing. ▶ Loosen your grip on the ball.

Power Jacks

Beginner: Follow the directions below.

Intermediate: Clap your hands once high above your head then again at chest level before catching the ball.

Advanced: Clap your hands behind your head once, then at chest level before chasing the ball downward and catching it.

Emphasizes: Chest, shoulders, lower back, hips, and legs.

Functional improvements: Improves concentration, proprioception, reaction time, and functional strength; prevents lower back and hip stiffness or injuries.

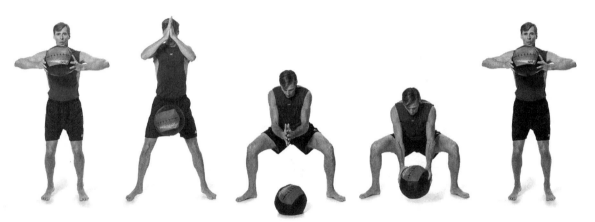

Begin with your feet parallel but farther than shoulder-width apart. Hold the ball in front of your chest with your elbows pointed outward.

Drop the ball, and a split second after you release it, quickly squat straight down so that you "follow" the ball downward as it falls. After the ball bounces, clap your hands once and catch it, then stand up straight while holding the ball in front of your face with your elbows out. Going down and up completes one repetition. Exhale when you squat and when you stand up.

DO:	DON'T:
▶ Begin with a wide stance.	▶ Lose your balance.
▶ Squat straight down.	▶ Cheat on the hand clap.
▶ Hold the ball in the proper position as you rise.	
▶ Lean over to grab the ball.	

Dough Kneading

Beginner: Slowly rotate your body entirely around in a 360-degree circle as you're kneading the ball. For your second set, rotate in the opposite direction.

Intermediate: Balance on one leg while you knead the ball. For your second set, switch legs.

Advanced: Balance on one leg and rotate 360 degrees while you knead the ball. Switch legs and rotate in the opposite direction for your second set.

Emphasizes: Fingers, wrists, forearms, upper arms, chest, shoulders, and core muscles.

Functional improvements: Prevents injuries in hands, fingers, wrists, and elbows; relieves sore joints in hands; improves grip; and improves consistency in swinging a golf club or tennis racket.

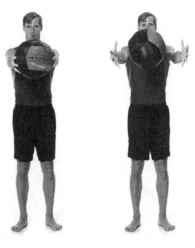

Begin with your feet in a parallel stance. Hold the ball in front of your chest with your arms extended.

Release the ball for a split second and grab it again, digging your fingertips and palms deeply into it. Quickly do this over and over as if you're vigorously kneading a ball of dough. Focus on your "suck and tuck" posture. Exhale each time you catch the ball.

DO:

▶ Hold the ball at chest level.

DON'T:

▶ Let your arms sag.
▶ Actually drop the ball when you release it. You should grab it quickly without letting it fall.

Spider Walk

Beginner: Follow the directions below.

Intermediate: Push the ball farther away.

Advanced: Roll the ball out to the left, then behind your legs, then out to the right so that the path forms an arch behind you. Go back and forth this way. Also, keep your eyes closed.

Emphasizes: Hamstrings, lower back, buttocks, inner and outer thighs, core muscles, shoulders.

Functional improvements: Relieves stiffness in the lower back and hips; strengthens and protects knees; prevents groin injuries; makes squatting and lifting objects easier; improves balance and control on uneven or slippery surfaces; makes climbing ladders and stairs easier; improves jumping and leaping; functionally strengthens lower extremities.

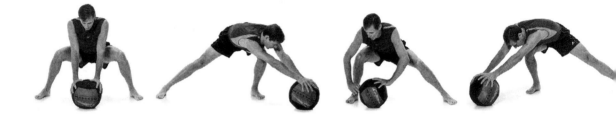

Begin with your feet in a parallel stance but spaced more than shoulder-width apart. Set the ball on the floor so that you're straddling it, and place both hands on the ball. Bend your knees and lower your buttocks until your thighs are parallel to the floor, and dig into the floor with your big toes.

With both hands, roll the ball out to the left away from you as far as you can go. Roll it back to the center, then out to the right to complete one repetition. Take two breaths while rolling the ball in each direction.

DO:

- ► Lean over but keep your back straight.
- ► Keep your buttocks low to the floor.
- ► Keep your head aligned with your spine.

DON'T:

- ► Hunch over.
- ► Use only one hand. Try to keep both hands on the ball as much as possible.
- ► Rest your body weight on the ball.
- ► Roll your feet over.

Progressive Cycles Move You to Success

Behind-the-Leg Pass

Emphasizes: Upper body, core muscles, thighs, and hamstrings.

Functional improvements: Improves balance, coordination, and quickness; lengthens strides and makes them more powerful and efficient; prevents hamstring and lower back injuries; makes climbing easier; improves your ability to multitask.

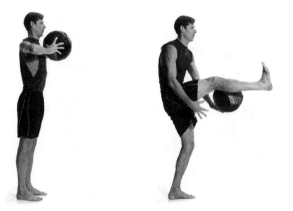

Begin with your feet parallel and spaced a few inches apart. Hold the ball in front of your chest with your elbows pointed outward.

Lift your leg straight up and pass the ball under your leg. The ball should travel to the outside of your thigh, under, back up past your inner thigh, and end in both hands above your leg again. Lower your leg to the starting position to complete the repetition. Do this in one smooth motion—imagine a basketball player passing the ball under his leg. Exhale when you pass the ball under your leg. Complete all the repetitions with one leg, then repeat with the other.

DO:	DON'T:
▶ Keep your leg straight as you bring it up.	▶ Lean or hunch over.
▶ Use steady, controlled movements.	▶ Swing your moving leg behind your standing leg.
▶ Keep your back straight.	▶ Bend your knees.

Twist and Sweep

Beginner: Look straight ahead during the motion.

Intermediate: Turn your head toward the direction of the ball's motion.

Advanced: Turn your head in the opposite direction of the ball's motion.

Emphasizes: Chest, shoulders, core muscles, waist, lower back, the adductor and abductor muscles of your thighs, and ankle stabilizers.

Benefits: Improves dynamic balance in walking or running; increases mobility of the neck, upper body, waist, lower back, and hips; reduces injuries to thighs or hips; strengthens ankles and feet for dynamic activities and sports; improves awareness of alignment and good posture; and flattens the abdominals to support the lower back.

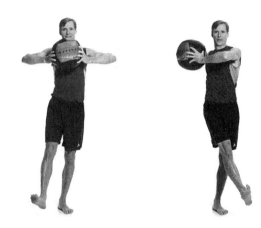

Start by standing on your left foot, with your right foot lifted a few inches in front of you, your toes pointed. Hold the ball in front of your chest with your elbows pointing outward.

Twist your upper chest (and the ball) to the right while sweeping your right foot to the left. Your pelvis stays stationary and your abdominals and lower back control the motion—but only your chest and leg are moving.

During this motion, your standing leg remains straight and your foot stays pointed forward. Imagine putting a golf ball with your instep, then with the outer edge of your foot, as your lifted foot sweeps from side to side. Breathe out as you twist in either direction. Complete all repetitions on one side, then switch sides.

DO:

▶ Move in a controlled motion.

▶ Lead slightly with your heel when moving your foot.

▶ Only move your foot back and forth as far as it will go without shifting your hips.

DON'T:

▶ Let your standing foot wobble—it should point forward the entire time.

▶ Sweep your leg so far that it causes your hips to turn.

▶ Bend your sweeping leg.

Progressive Cycles Move You to Success

CYCLE TWO CHART

	WEEK 1 15 to 20 min each program	WEEK 2 20 to 25 min each program	WEEK 3 25 to 35 min each program	WEEK 4 35 to 45 min each program
The Coil, each direction	4 first session 6 second session 8 third session	6 first session 8 second session 10 third session	8 first session 10 second session 12 third session	10 first session 12 second session 15 third session
Advanced Push and Pull, each side	5 6 8	6 8 10	8 12 15	12 15 20
Diagonal Chop, each direction	5 6 8	7 8 10	9 10 12	10 12 15

Do a second set of the first three techniques, then move to the second group of four.

Golfer Swing, each side	5 6 10	8 10 15	10 14 20	12 16 25
Statue of Liberty, each side	5 6 10	7 9 12	9 12 15	12 15 20
Power Jacks	5 7 10	8 9 12	10 12 15	12 15 20
Dough Kneading	5 8 10	8 10 12	10 12 15	12 15 20

Do a second set of the middle four techniques, then move to the last group of three.

Spider Walk, each side	4 6 8	6 8 10	8 10 12	10 12 15
Behind-the-Leg Pass, each side	4 6 8	6 8 10	8 12 15	10 15 20
Twist and Sweep, each side	6 8 10	8 10 12	10 12 15	12 15 20

Do a second set of the final three techniques, then move to the relaxation/stretching techniques below. (See pages 41 to 43.)

Wedge

Lying Side Twist

Spread Eagle

5

THE THIRD CYCLE

As you progress through this third month, you should become more comfortable with your body's movements. Your muscles are growing stronger and more flexible. Your confidence level has increased and you are lighter on your feet.

Moving has become easier. You feel taller, and your posture is improving. You feel more at ease moving your arms and legs because your joints' range of motion has improved. If you play sports, you likely feel more coordinated, with a faster reaction time.

You should have more energy to perform your daily activities, and you should be sleeping better. Prior to starting this program, if you regularly had morning stiffness, that should have improved or gone away.

Some of the activities in the third month contain more challenging movements, while others take advantage of skills you've already mastered. However, you're well prepared at this point to take your body to the next level.

Knee Lift and Side Twist

Beginner: Look straight ahead during the motion, and touch your foot to the floor between repetitions.

Intermediate: Look straight ahead, but keep your thigh raised throughout the movement, not touching your foot to the floor between repetitions.

Advanced: Turn your head along with your torso during the twist, and keep your thigh raised throughout the movement, not touching your foot to the floor between repetitions.

Emphasizes: Shoulders, chest, upper and lower back, core muscles, hips, and thighs.

Functional improvements: Helps lower your likelihood of dizziness; improves ability to twist your torso while moving; improves peripheral vision and balance; lengthens your stride; alleviates or eliminates hip and back pain; improves your ability to multitask; establishes body symmetry; decreases swaying of the hips or swinging of the legs; and reduces wear and tear on joints.

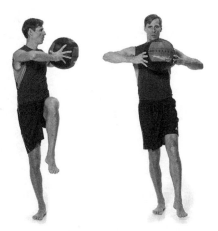

Start with your feet parallel and closer than shoulder-width apart. Hold the ball in front of your chest with your elbows pointing out to the side.

Twist your torso all the way to the left while you raise your left thigh until it's parallel with the floor.

As you set your foot back down, twist your torso all the way to the right. Return your torso to center to complete the repetition. Breathe out as you twist in each direction.

DO:

▶ Twist as far as you can to each side.
▶ Maintain good posture throughout the motion.
▶ Keep your arms and legs moving at the same speed.

DON'T:

▶ Lean back.
▶ Lift the heel of your standing foot off of the floor.
▶ Bend your standing leg.
▶ Relax your fingers or thumbs.
▶ Lower the ball and your arms below chest level.

Carioca Loop

Beginner: Follow the directions below.

Intermediate: At the end of the motion, drop the ball and catch it after one bounce.

Advanced: At the end of the motion, drop the ball, clap your hands, and catch it after one bounce.

Emphasizes: The entire body, with extra focus on the shoulder girdle, arms, core muscles, buttocks, and inner and outer thighs.

Functional improvements: Improves dynamic balance and coordination; increases your ability to carry a load; strengthens and loosens hips; helps prevent groin or hip injuries; strengthens the cardiopulmonary system; improves your rhythm; improves side-to-side movements; improves the ability to lift or squat while twisting or turning; and improves your core function and resilience.

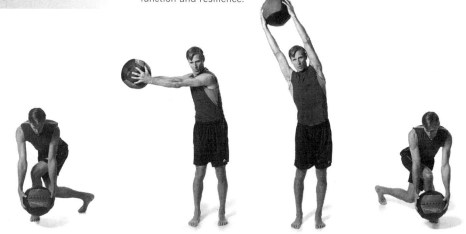

Begin by squatting down with most of your weight on your left leg, and your right foot touching the floor behind you and out to your left. Both knees should be bent and your right foot should be resting on the ball of the foot. Lean forward, fully extend your arms, and let the ball hang past your left knee.

Keeping your arms fully extended, bring the ball in a wide circle toward the right, then overhead, while at the same time stepping up with your back foot into a parallel stance. You should reach this stance just as the ball reaches the point straight overhead. Continue moving the ball in a circle toward the left and down as you step behind with your left foot. You will end up with most of your weight on your right leg, with your left leg behind you and out to your right, and your arms fully extended and holding the ball just below your right knee. This is the mirror opposite of how you started. Complete all repetitions in this direction, then switch directions and repeat.

Exhale while you're lifting and lowering the ball.

DO:

▶ Make sure your back foot is pressed firmly to the floor.

▶ Keep your back straight, and bend from the waist at the beginning and end.

▶ Reach out with your arms as far as you can to make the circle as wide as possible.

▶ Make one continuous motion without any stops.

DON'T:

▶ Hunch over at the beginning and end.

▶ Loosen your grip on the ball.

Progressive Cycles Move You to Success

Straddle Squat and Reach

Beginner: Finish with the ball in front of your chest.

Intermediate: Finish with the ball angled toward the ceiling.

Advanced: Finish with the ball overhead, then toss it into the air and catch it.

Emphasizes: Shoulders, back, buttocks, inner thighs, and core muscles.

Functional improvements: Stretches and strengthens your lower back; gives you a farther reach; allows you to pick up heavier items; improves spatial awareness and dynamic balance; improves the ability to shift directions quickly; and improves stability in walking and running activities.

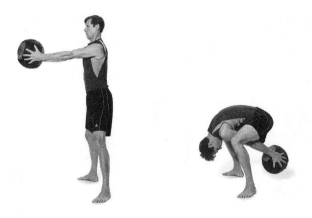

Begin with your feet parallel but spaced very far apart. Your toes should be pointed outward. Press your big toes into the floor. Hold the ball at arm's length in front of your chest with both hands.

Squat down, lean forward, and push the ball between your legs as far back as possible. This time, allow your entire back to become rounded as you push the ball, so that you feel a good stretch in your lower back.

Exhale as you reach down, again as you hold the final position, and again as you stand up. Return to the starting point to finish the repetition.

DO:

▶ Start with your feet wider than shoulder-width apart.

▶ Point your toes outward.

DON'T:

▶ Let your knees buckle inward. They should point over the toes.

▶ Limit your reach through the legs. Reach as far as you can for better back mobility.

▶ Just bend with your lower back.

Atlas

Beginner: Follow the directions below.

Intermediate: After you catch the ball, change the direction you bring it around to your front (left, right, left). Also, close your eyes.

Advanced: Stand on one leg, but keep your eyes open.

Emphasizes: Neck, arms and shoulders, upper and lower back, hips, and core muscles.

Functional improvements: Reduces risk of injury when bending over or carrying a load; improves kinesthetic awareness, posture, and proper alignment; improves reaction time; strengthens hands and provides more control while holding a weight or sports equipment.

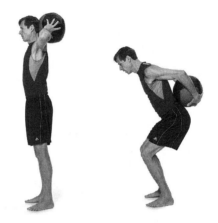

This movement requires quick motions. Begin with your feet parallel and spaced just a few inches apart. Hold the ball against the back of your neck with both hands. Squat down and lean forward slightly, while keeping your back straight. Your head should be in line with your back, not craned back or forward.

Release the ball, then immediately move your hands so that you're reaching behind your lower back, and catch the ball when it arrives. The ball should roll smoothly between your shoulder blades and down your back, with no bouncing. To make the ball roll more slowly, lean forward farther.

When you catch the ball, bring it back around to your front, then resume the starting position. Exhale three times during the exercise: when the ball rolls down your spine, when you catch it, and when you place it behind your head.

DO:

▶ Keep your back straight.

▶ Get ready to catch the ball as soon as you release it.

DON'T:

▶ Arch your back or hunch forward.

Thigh Kick and Soldier Walk

Beginner: Plant your foot on the floor after each repetition.

Intermediate: Only tap the floor with your foot after each repetition.

Advanced: Don't touch the floor with your foot until all repetitions are completed.

Emphasizes: Chest, shoulders, hands, hip flexors, thighs, hamstrings, and core muscles.

Functional improvements: Improves balance; strengthens ankles and feet; builds stamina; prevents injuries in the feet, hamstrings, and lower back; relieves stiffness and tightness in the hips and back; makes climbing stairs and ladders easier; sharpens the mind and body; and increases lung capacity through rhythmic breathing.

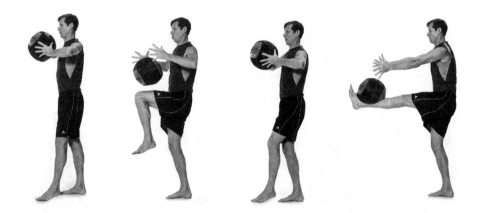

Begin with one foot extended, toes touching the floor. Hold the ball in front of your chest with your elbows pointing outward.

Lift the thigh of your extended leg until it's parallel with the floor, then drop the ball so that it bounces off your thigh. Grab the ball with both hands.

Lower your leg, then lift it again, this time fully extended in a soft lock. At the same time, extend your arms fully in front of your chest. As your shin comes up, drop the ball a few inches so that it taps your shin, and catch the ball with both hands. Lower your leg to complete the repetition. Exhale with each thigh lift and with each reach and catch. Complete all the repetitions using one foot, then switch feet and repeat.

DO:

▶ Maintain a straight, upright back while lifting your thigh, then your entire leg.

▶ Raise your leg in a smooth motion.

▶ Bend from your hips when you touch the ball to your shin.

▶ Keep your swinging leg as straight as possible.

DON'T:

▶ Make jerking motions.

▶ Hunch over when reaching the ball out to touch your shin.

▶ Kick hard or touch your knee.

Overhead Juggling

Beginner: Follow the directions below.

Intermediate: Begin with your feet together. As the ball passes overhead, step out with one foot. As you lower your arms down to your sides, bring your second foot out to join the one you just moved.

Advanced: Start in a deep parallel stance and take three shuffle steps to one side as the ball goes overhead.

Emphasizes: The entire body with a focus on the arms, hands and fingers, shoulders and neck, outer thighs, knees, ankles, and core muscles.

Functional improvements: Strengthens the entire shoulder girdle proportionally; improves dynamic flexibility in the shoulders; strengthens the hands; gives better balance and body control when moving sideways; strengthens the ankles; improves agility, peripheral vision, and spatial awareness; increases kinesthetic awareness of the body in motion; and strengthens the cardiopulmonary system.

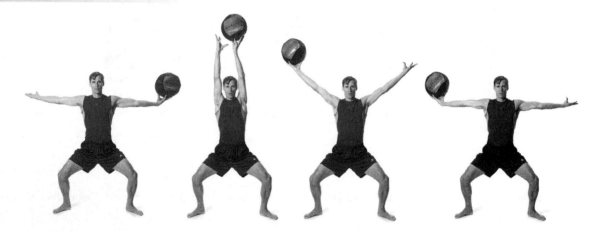

Begin with your feet parallel but spaced wider than shoulder-width apart. Your toes should be pointed outward. Squat down with your arms fully extended to your sides, with the ball in one hand.

Move both arms straight overhead and pass the ball to your other hand. Bring your arms back out to your sides while keeping your arms extended. The ball will end up on the opposite side from where it started. Exhale with each overhead pass. Complete all repetitions in one direction, then switch directions and repeat.

DO:

▶ Grip the ball tightly with your fingertips, but also keep it balanced in your hand.

DON'T:

▶ Lean or hunch forward while moving your arms.
▶ Juggle the ball in front of you.

Around the World

Emphasizes: The feet, hips, back, hamstrings, thighs, arms, shoulders, and core muscles.

Functional improvements: Improves balance and stability; creates better shoulder flexibility and reach; strengthens the knees and feet; strengthens and lengthens the inner thigh muscles; improves back flexibility; relieves tension and stiffness throughout the body; lengthens your stride; improves your equilibrium, peripheral vision, and spatial awareness; and strengthens muscle groups in your back.

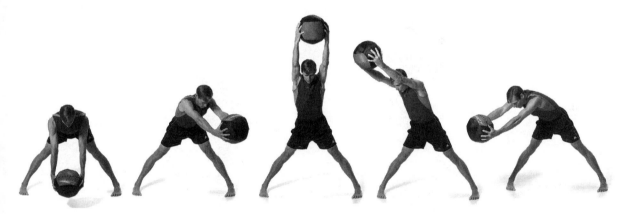

Begin with your feet in a parallel stance, spaced farther than shoulder-width apart. Keep your legs straight, with your toes pointed inward and pressed into the floor. Lean forward deeply and hold the ball toward the floor in both hands with your arms fully extended.

Reaching out as far as you can, move the ball out to your left and up until it's overhead, and on to your right and back down to the starting point. As you reach the high point of this circle, stretch yourself up as tall as you can. Keep your arms and legs straight as you make the circle. Finish all the repetitions in one direction, then switch directions.

Exhale as your hands travel past each quarter of the circle.

DO:

► Keep your stance deep and your toes pointed inward.

► Bend from the waist as you lean over.

► Use fluid motions.

DON'T:

► Slouch or round your shoulders as you move through the bottom portion of the circle.

► Bend at the knees.

► Stop breathing.

Leg Extension Opposite Reach

Beginner: Follow the directions below.

Intermediate: Hold your thigh parallel with the floor during the entire motion. Do not touch the floor.

Advanced: Follow the intermediate instructions, but pivot a few degrees on your foot after each repetition so you complete a 360-degree circle.

Emphasizes: The chest, shoulders, upper back, thighs, hamstrings, rotator cuffs, and core muscles.

Functional improvements: Improves balance and coordination when multitasking; builds core and shoulder stability; improves your arm reach; lengthens and strengthens your thighs and arms; increases ankle and foot strength; and increases stamina.

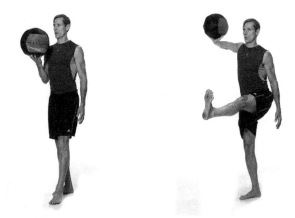

Stand with most of your weight on your right foot, with your left foot resting on the floor a few inches in front of you. Hold the ball in your right hand in front of your chest, with your elbow bent.

Bring the ball out to your right side until your arm is fully extended. While you are reaching with your arm, lift your left thigh until it's parallel to the floor, and extend your leg out in front of you as far as you can. Return your arm to the starting position, lowering your leg to complete the repetition. Complete all the repetitions on the right side, then switch sides.

Breathe out while you're reaching your hand out, and again when you pull it back.

DO:	DON'T:
▶ Hold your back upright.	▶ Hunch over.
▶ Look forward during the entire move.	▶ Move one limb first and then the other. Move them in unison.
▶ Suck your belly in.	▶ Rest with your weight on the heel of your back foot. Place the emphasis and pressure on the ball of your standing foot.

Mower

Emphasizes: The shoulders, hands, fingers, neck, chest, triceps, all the core muscles, and the lats.

Functional improvements: Improves your awareness of body alignment, balance and posture; increases neck, shoulder, and torso flexibility; improves equilibrium; makes twisting and reaching easier; improves peripheral vision; flattens the abdominals; and strengthens hip, knee, and ankle stabilizers.

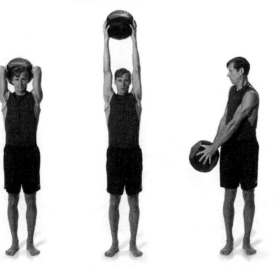

Begin in a parallel stance with your feet a few inches apart. Hold the ball in both hands behind the back of your neck, keeping your upper arms close to your ears.

Reach up and extend your arms overhead into a soft lock, then bring the ball down to one side until your upper body has twisted in that direction to complete one repetition. Keep your arms fully extended and do not shrug your shoulders upward. Switch sides for each repetition.

Exhale when you lower the ball and again when you lift your arms.

DO:

▶ Hold your hips steady—the twisting motion as you bring the ball down to your side should come from your abdominals and your lower back muscles.

▶ Lean over slightly as the ball comes down to your side.

▶ Grip the floor with your toes when turning.

DON'T:

▶ Slouch or hunch.

▶ Twist your knees.

▶ Arch backward.

Split Stand Reach to Toes

Beginner: Begin with your feet in a relatively close stance.

Intermediate: Widen your stance and reach out farther with the ball.

Advanced: Start in as wide a stance as possible.

Emphasizes: The hamstrings, calves, core muscles, and upper back.

Functional improvements: Improves dynamic balance; strengthens the muscles in the groin, knees, and feet to better align your legs; improves walking, running, and sprinting abilities; reduces risk of injuries; gives functional strength to the lower back and hamstrings; improves reaching and lifting ability; and improves kinesthetic awareness.

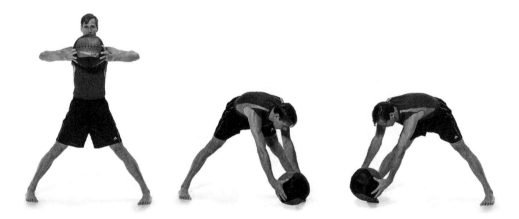

Begin in a wide parallel stance with your legs straight and your toes pointed inward. Hold the ball to your chest with your elbows pointed outward.

Lean forward and, with your arms fully extended, try to touch one foot with the ball. If you're more flexible, reach out even farther. Stand back up and pull the ball to your chest to complete the repetition. Complete all the repetitions on one side, then switch sides and repeat.

Breathe out when you reach down and again when you lift yourself up.

DO:

▶ Turn your entire upper body toward the desired direction.

▶ Return to a fully upright position between repetitions.

▶ Keep your weight on the balls of your feet.

DON'T:

▶ Let your legs slide apart.

CYCLE THREE CHART

	WEEK 1 15 to 20 min each program	WEEK 2 20 to 25 min each program	WEEK 3 25 to 35 min each program	WEEK 4 35 to 45 min each program
Knee Lift and Side Twist, each side	5 first session 6 second session 8 third session	7 first session 9 second session 10 third session	10 first session 12 second session 15 third session	12 first session 15 second session 20 third session
Carioca Loop, each direction	5 7 10	7 9 12	9 12 15	12 15 20
Straddle Squat and Reach	6 8 10	8 10 12	10 12 15	12 15 20

Do a second set of the first three techniques, then move to the second group of four.

Atlas, each side	6 8 10	8 10 12	10 12 15	12 15 20
Thigh Kick and Soldier Walk, each leg	5 7 9	7 9 12	9 12 15	12 15 20
Overhead Juggling, each side	5 7 10	7 9 12	9 12 15	12 15 20
Around the World, each direction	4 6 8	6 8 10	8 10 12	10 12 15

Do a second set of the middle four techniques, then move to the last group of three.

Leg Extension Opposite Reach, each side	5 8 10	6 10 12	8 12 15	10 15 20
Mower, each side	4 6 8	6 8 12	8 12 15	10 15 20
Split Stand Reach to Toes, each side	4 6 8	6 8 12	8 12 15	10 15 20

Do a second set of the final three techniques, then move to the relaxation/stretching techniques below. (See pages 41 to 43.)

Wedge

Lying Side Twist

Spread Eagle

6

THE FOURTH CYCLE

You've reached the final monthlong cycle of the program. You'll find that these movements are even more challenging than those you've done in earlier cycles, though some build upon skills you've already learned.

Your muscles require time to grow strong—at least 4 months of progressively increasing challenge. Other skills, such as flexibility, also require this much time. Changing the techniques you perform every 4 weeks keeps changing the challenge to your muscles, which causes them to respond by growing stronger.

You're almost to the end of the program, and I hope you're able to see many improvements in the way your body functions. The final total mind and body technique this month is the granddaddy of all the *Four Way Burn* activities. It's called Way Down and Way Up, and it will require complete control over your body—and a fair amount of patience—to get it right.

Good Morning with Side Twist

Beginner: Do as directed below.

Intermediate: Cross your legs and place your feet side by side. When your left foot is crossed over the right, twist your torso to the left, and vice versa.

Advanced: Perform the moves with your eyes closed and your feet in a split stance (one in front, one in back, and spaced shoulder-width apart).

Emphasizes: The core muscles, lower back, waist, trunk, hamstrings, hips, buttocks, and shoulders.

Functional improvements: Reduces and prevents morning stiffness in the lower back; improves functional abdominal strength; creates more neck and upper body flexibility; improves equilibrium; prevents lower back and hamstring pulls; improves functional mobility while moving; creates greater ease in bending down to pick things up.

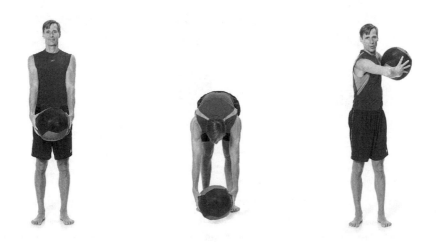

Begin with your feet parallel and closer than shoulder-width apart. At the starting position, hold the ball downward in front of your groin with your arms fully extended.

Lean straight down and touch the ball to the floor in front of your feet. Now, stand up while bringing the ball to your chest, and fully twist your torso to one side. While twisting, make sure that your elbows don't drop below chest level. Return your torso so that you're facing center to complete the repetition. Alternate between twisting left and right with each repetition. Exhale as you bend down and as you twist.

DO:

▶ Stand up straight before twisting your torso.

▶ Move only your torso as you twist, not your hips.

DON'T:

▶ Stop between the Good Morning portion and the Side Twist.

▶ Overtwist.

Race Car Driver

Emphasizes: The shoulders, arms, chest, core muscles, and hips.

Functional improvements: Strengthens the hands, elbows, and arms; creates resilience and mental toughness; reestablishes a strong bridge between the shoulder girdle and the lower body; improves alignment and posture awareness; prevents tennis elbow and carpal tunnel syndrome; tightens and flattens the abdominals to support the lower back when sitting, walking, or jogging; improves your ability to multitask.

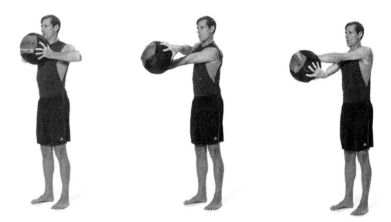

Begin in a parallel stance, standing tall with your feet a few inches apart. Hold the ball between both hands at your chest. Extend your arms in a soft lock in front of your chest. Your hands should be placed at the left and right sides of the ball. Counter the weight you are holding, and keep from arching your back, by "sucking and tucking" your pelvis.

Now, twist the ball between your hands as if you're turning a steering wheel. Your arms may touch if you twist the ball far enough, but only twist as far as you can while keeping your shoulders square. When you have twisted as far as you comfortably can in one direction, twist to the other direction to complete one repetition. Exhale with each rotation.

DO:	DON'T:
▶ Squeeze the ball tightly.	▶ Shrug up your shoulders.
▶ Keep both arms straight at all times.	▶ Lower your arms before the set is completed.

Progressive Cycles Move You to Success

Pecking Bird

Emphasizes: The hips, thighs, feet, core muscles.

Functional improvements: Strengthens both hips and legs equally; creates more strength, control, and power when walking, jogging, and sprinting; makes climbing easier; improves your balance while bending down; reduces hip or lower back problems; strengthens the feet, ankles, and Achilles tendons; improves equilibrium; and improves cardiopulmonary efficiency.

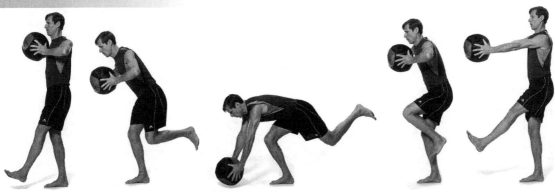

Stand on one foot, with your other leg extended in front of you and its foot raised a few inches off the floor. Hold the ball at chest level with your elbows pointed out.

Slowly lean forward, extend your arms, and touch the ball to the floor (or reach as far as you can). As you're leaning over, do a mini-squat on your standing leg, and bring your front leg back behind you, bending it at the knee.

Straighten back up and push the ball out at chest level, simultaneously bringing your rear leg back out to the front. Momentarily recover at your starting position, then repeat until you have completed all repetitions on that leg. Then switch legs and repeat.

Exhale four times—when you lean and squat down, when you stand back up, when you push the ball out, and when you pull it back to your chest.

DO:	DON'T:
▶ Move in a careful, controlled manner.	▶ Touch the floor with your raised leg.
▶ Stop if the motion hurts your knee. Refrain from doing this technique if you have knee pain. It indicates that the leg is not strong enough to support your entire weight on one knee.	▶ Lose your balance.
▶ Keep your back as straight as possible.	

Figure Eight Walk

Beginner: Spread your feet only as far as is comfortable.

Intermediate: Spread your feet in a wider stance.

Advanced: Spread your feet farther apart and keep your eyes closed.

Emphasizes: The hamstrings, lower back, hips, thighs, and core muscles.

Functional improvements: Strengthens the lower back, buttocks, and thighs proportionately; makes squatting easier; helps you leap forward and sideways; improves your cardiopulmonary system; relieves and protects the lower back; removes tightness around the hips, inner thighs, and groin; improves reaction time, agility, and stamina; and improves your balance on wet and slippery surfaces.

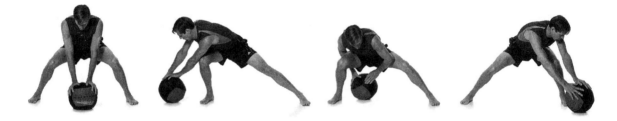

Begin in a wide parallel stance, with your feet spaced as far apart as you can comfortably get them. Lean forward and place the ball on the floor in front of you.

Pushing the ball with both hands, roll it around and between your legs so that its path forms a figure eight around your feet. Shift your upper body as you move the ball so that your chest stays pointed at the ball throughout its movement. Push your body toward the direction you are passing the ball, to improve your reach. When you have completed the passes in one direction, repeat, moving the ball in the opposite direction.

Take four breaths for each figure eight pass. Breathe out as the ball goes behind and in front of each leg as you're rolling it around your legs.

DO:

▶ Stretch yourself out as far as possible while moving the ball.

DON'T:

▶ Just use one hand to roll the ball—use both.

▶ Let your feet roll out onto their edges. Press the insides of your feet down into the floor.

Triceps and Leg Extensions

Emphasizes: The triceps, shoulders, core muscles, abdominals, thighs, hamstrings, and feet.

Functional improvements: Improves alignment, balance, and posture; improves overhead reach; strengthens and flattens abdominals to align the pelvis, relieving lower back pain and stiffness; strengthens the hips and legs proportionally; strengthens the muscles around the knees, and your ankles and feet, protecting them from injuries; and increases proprioception and kinesthetic awareness.

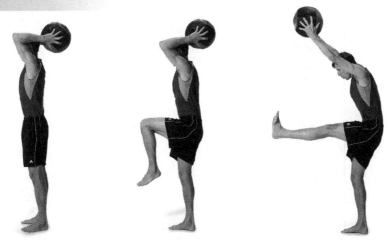

Begin in a parallel stance with your feet just a few inches apart. "Suck and tuck" your pelvis. Hold the ball with both hands behind the back of your neck, keeping your elbows close to your head.

Lift one leg until your thigh is parallel with the floor, and extend your foot until your leg is straight. You should feel the stretch behind your thigh. At the same time, bring the ball over your head and forward until your arms are fully extended at an upward angle toward the ceiling. Return to the starting position to complete the repetition. Alternate feet with each repetition. Exhale when you reach out with the ball and again when you pull it back.

DO:

▶ Keep your back upright during the motion.

▶ Extend your leg far enough so that you feel a soft lock in the knee.

DON'T:

▶ Crane your head down while bringing the ball over your head—keep looking forward.

▶ Round your shoulders.

▶ Stop breathing rhythmically.

Crescent Reach

Emphasizes: The hips, waist, neck and lat muscles, front shoulder girdle, rotator cuffs, core muscles, hands, arms, and shoulders.

Functional improvements: Improves awareness of body alignment and balance; makes you feel taller; makes reaching overhead and to the sides easier; prevents injuries in rotator cuffs and shoulders; tightens and flattens abdominal muscles; reduces and prevents hip and waist stiffness; strengthens hands and fingers.

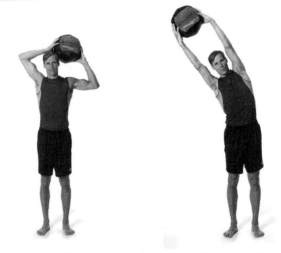

Begin in a parallel stance with a tall posture, your feet a few inches apart. Hold the ball firmly between your hands above your left shoulder. Your elbows should be pointed outward.

Fully extend your arms upward and at an angle to the right while tilting your upper body to the right. Your arms should be alongside your head, not in front of it or behind it. Visualize your body shaped like a crescent moon.

Return your torso to center and lower the ball back to your shoulder, lowering your elbows down toward the floor, to complete the repetition. Exhale when you push the ball upward and again when you bring it back down. After you've completed the repetitions to the right, repeat to the left.

DO:	DON'T:
▶ Hold your hips steady and bend from the waist. ▶ Feel your body weight over the balls of your feet.	▶ Push your hip out in the opposite direction from your motion. ▶ Hunch forward. ▶ Relax your abdominal muscles.

Knee Tuck and Push

Beginner: Follow the directions below.

Intermediate: Stand on one foot during the entire activity.

Advanced: Follow the intermediate directions, but pivot on your standing leg a few degrees with each repetition so that you turn in a 360-degree circle.

Emphasizes: The hips, thighs, back, hamstrings, chest, shoulder girdle, core muscles, and feet.

Functional improvements: Improves lower back mobility; strengthens the rear shoulder girdle; improves posture and balance; improves your ability to reach and pull while in motion; strengthens the hips and hip flexors for easier walking and climbing; improves foot strength and mind-body connection so you can walk better on uneven ground; and increases your awareness of the muscles in your back.

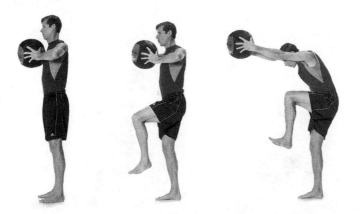

Begin in a parallel stance with your feet a few inches apart, while holding the ball in front of your chest with your elbows pointed outward.

Lift one thigh upward until it's higher than parallel with the floor, keeping your foot flexed. At the same time, lean your upper body forward and extend your arms in a soft lock so that the ball is held out from your body. It's okay to lower your head and hunch forward as you press the ball outward. Put your weight on the ball of the foot on which you're standing.

To complete the repetition, lower your foot and straighten that leg. Stand upright, and bring the ball back to your chest, keeping your elbows between chest and shoulder height and pulling your shoulder blades together. Exhale once as you push the ball away from you and again as you pull it back. Complete all repetitions on one side, then switch sides and repeat.

DO:

▶ Lift your thigh up as high as you can.

▶ Extend your arms fully when you lean forward.

▶ Suck in your abdominals when you lean forward.

DON'T:

▶ Hold your breath.

▶ Loosen your grip on the ball.

▶ Lift one leg higher or lower than the other.

Back Lunge with Double Twist and Kick

Beginner: Bend your rear knee moderately when you are in the lunge position.

Intermediate: Increase your stride and lower your rear knee closer to the floor, but keep your leg straight.

Advanced: Follow the intermediate directions, but keep your eyes closed.

Emphasizes: The legs, feet, hips, front and rear shoulder girdle, and core muscles.

Functional improvements: Improves dynamic balance and lateral stability; strengthens and supports the front, side, and back of the knees; increases kinesthetic awareness; improves functional abdominal strength; strengthens hamstrings, internal hip rotators, and buttocks, giving your legs stability and support for walking and running; reduces the risk of injury to your knees, hips, and back; increases your range of mobility when twisting from side to side; improves peripheral vision and spatial awareness; increases stride length for a more powerful walk or run; and enhances the cardiovascular system.

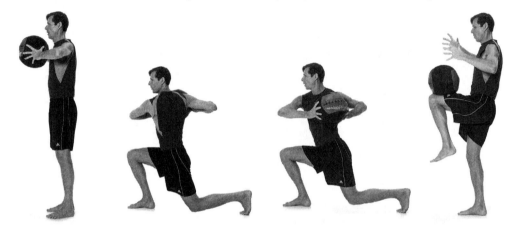

Begin in a parallel stance with your feet a few inches apart, holding the ball in front of your chest with your elbows out. Extend one leg behind you, keeping your knee off the floor so that your foot is resting on the toes and ball of the foot. It's as if you're taking a long step backward. Keep your weight centered.

Once in position, twist your torso in one direction, then the other. Don't lower the ball or let your elbows drop beneath your chest.

Bring your back leg up in front of you until your thigh is parallel with the floor. Drop the ball so that it bounces off your knee. Return to the lunge position to begin the next repetition. Exhale four times—when you lunge back, when you twist to one side and then the other, and when you bounce the ball off your thigh. Complete all your repetitions with one leg, then repeat with the other leg.

DO:

▶ Hold the ball at chest height.
▶ Keep your front knee aligned with your foot.

DON'T:

▶ Let your back knee and foot become twisted.
▶ Lean over.
▶ Arch backward.

Front-Arm Raise with Leg Abduction

Beginner: Set your foot back on the floor after each repetition.

Intermediate: Only touch your toes to the floor between repetitions.

Advanced: Don't touch the floor between repetitions. Also, when you lift the ball, toss it up a few inches and catch it.

Emphasizes: The arms, shoulders and shoulder girdle, core muscles, abdominals, waist, hips, inner and outer thighs, knee stabilizers, and feet.

Functional improvements: Improves lateral hip stability and dynamic balance for walking and running activities; prevents hip stiffness; improves posture; increases your ability to move laterally; increases functional abdominal and lower back strength; decreases the risk of ankle and foot injury; and improves coordination.

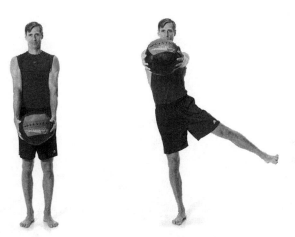

Stand in a parallel stance with your feet shoulder-width apart. Hold the ball in both hands with a strong grip and your arms fully extended so that the ball is in front of your groin.

Lift one leg out to the side while lifting the ball upward until your arms are parallel to the floor, keeping your arms and legs fully extended. To complete the repetition, lower your arms to the starting position and lower your foot until your heels touch. Complete all repetitions, then switch sides and repeat.

Exhale when lifting the ball and again when lowering it.

DO:

▶ Extend your leg outward as far as you can without having to pivot your hips. Your hips should remain motionless.

▶ Pull in your abdominal muscles.

DON'T:

▶ Raise your leg so far that you have to lean back or turn your hips to go higher.

Way Down and Way Up

Beginner: Follow the directions below.

Intermediate: Lie down in a different direction each time.

Advanced: Do this with your eyes closed.

Emphasizes: The entire body, particularly your core muscles.

Functional improvements: Enables you to better lift and lower yourself with ease from the floor, bed, or couch; reduces your risk of injury while falling; improves recovery time in athletic activities; improves spatial awareness, kinesthetic awareness, and dynamic balance; sharpens the mind and the body; and conditions the upper and lower body proportionally.

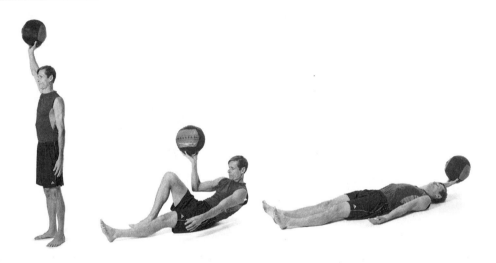

This will require a few more feet of floor space than the other activities; give yourself plenty of room on each side and overhead. Stand in a parallel stance with your feet a few inches apart, holding the ball in one hand as high as possible over your head.

Slowly lower the ball in front of you, allowing your arm to bend, and slowly lower your buttocks toward the floor. Sit down on the floor and lean back, all the while holding the ball aloft in the same hand.

Recline onto your back and extend the ball over your head until your arm is parallel with the floor and the ball is behind your head.

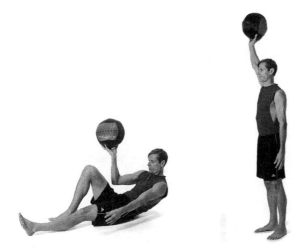

Slowly raise the ball, sit up, shift your weight to your hips and knees, and stand up. Return to the starting position to complete the repetition. Switch hands after each repetition.

Exhale four times as you go down, and four times as you lift yourself up. As you go to the floor, breathe as you bend over, squat down, sit down, and then lie down. On the way up, breathe as you lean forward, tuck your legs under you, stand up, and reach up.

DO:

▶ Complete the motion without using your empty hand for assistance while going to the floor and getting up, if possible.

▶ Allow your hand to rotate and pivot as you move to keep control of the ball.

DON'T:

▶ Lose control of the ball at any time.

When You've Finished the Fourth Month

Even when you complete the fourth cycle of *Four Way Burn*, your experience with the program is just beginning. You can choose from two options.

▶ You can begin a scaled-down version of the program that maintains your gains.

▶ You can begin the first cycle again, but make it more challenging in order to bump your fitness up another level.

Maintaining Your Improvements

If you want to sustain the improvements you've reaped from this program, you'll need to keep practicing the techniques. However, in this maintenance phase, you'll only need to do a handful of techniques.

Each day, choose five techniques that together include the following motions.

1. Standing on one leg
2. Bending over from the waist
3. Squatting
4. Pushing

5. Pulling
6. Twisting your upper body
7. Turning your entire body

You can choose whichever five techniques you want, as long as they provide all seven of these movements.

Try to find a group of five to do one day, and a different five the next day, and alternate between the techniques. Each day, do the first two techniques—15 reps each—then repeat for a second set. Then do 15 reps each of the next three techniques, and repeat those for a second set.

For example, the first three days might look like:

First Day	Second Day	Third Day
1. Side Twist	1. Knee Lift and Side Twist	1. Rocking Chair
2. Good Morning	2. Mower	2. Atlas
3. Squat and Push	3. Figure Eight Walk	3. Pecking Bird
4. Soldier Walk	4. The Coil	4. Race Car Driver
5. Saturn	5. Twist and Sweep	5. Way Down and Way Up

Taking It to the Next Level

The other alternative—if you want to challenge yourself even more at the end of the fourth cycle—is to make your sessions even tougher. One way to do this is to keep moving up the scale from beginner to advanced. Doing the program at all three levels will take a whole year.

At the end of the year, stick with the advanced level but try these 10 steps to make the program even more challenging and interesting.

1. Change the direction in which you are facing.

2. Change the room in which you do these activities.

3. Try to close your eyes.

4. Move outdoors and stand on a different surface, such as grass, dirt, a wooden deck, or concrete.

5. Change the weight you're holding from 4 to 5 or 6 pounds.

6. Rest for a shorter time—or take no rest—between each technique and set.

7. Use a metronome and follow a specific pace.

8. Stretch out your arms or legs for a farther reach while you're moving.

9. Move the ball faster or slower.

10. Squeeze the ball harder.

CYCLE FOUR CHART

	WEEK 1 20 to 25 min each program	WEEK 2 25 to 35 min each program	WEEK 3 35 to 40 min each program	WEEK 4 45 to 50 min each program
Good Morning with Side Twist, per side	6 first session 8 second session 10 third session	8 first session 10 second session 12 third session	10 first session 12 second session 15 third session	10 first session 15 second session 20 third session
Race Car Driver	5 6 8	7 8 10	10 12 15	12 15 20
Pecking Bird, each leg	3 5 8	5 8 10	7 10 12	10 12 15
Do a second set of the first three techniques, then move to the second group of four.				
Figure Eight Walk, each direction	3 5 8	5 8 10	8 10 12	10 12 15
Triceps and Leg Extensions, each leg	5 8 10	6 10 12	8 12 15	10 15 20
Crescent Reach, each side	6 8 10	8 10 12	10 12 15	12 15 20
Knee Tuck and Push, each side	6 8 10	8 10 12	10 12 15	12 15 20
Do a second set of the second group of four techniques, then move to the final group of three.				
Back Lunge with Double Twist and Kick, each leg	3 5 8	5 7 10	7 9 12	10 12 15
Front-Arm Raise with Leg Abduction, each side	5 6 8	7 9 12	9 12 15	12 15 20
Way Down and Way Up, each side	3 5 7	5 7 10	7 10 12	10 12 15
Do a second set of the final three techniques, then move to the relaxation/stretching techniques below. (See pages 41 to 43.)				

Wedge

Lying Side Twist

Spread Eagle

ADAPTING
FOUR WAY BURN
FOR YOUR
NEEDS

7

STAY ON TRACK
WHILE YOU'RE TRAVELING

Over the years, many clients have asked me to plan an exercise program for them to follow so they could maintain their fitness gains while on vacation or a business trip. I've probably designed hundreds of these travel programs, based on their specific needs and geared to their specific interests, over the years.

Maintaining your physical activity routines while you're away from home is a great goal. Your healthy habits will sustain the fitness level you've achieved so that it doesn't fade while you're traveling.

However, you need a high level of motivation to maintain the fitness program that you do at home—especially with the same level of intensity—while you're on the road. Any travel program has to overcome a number of challenges.

First, the simple act of traveling requires lots of time and energy. You don't have as much of either to devote to your fitness.

Second, your stress level is high—even if you're on a pleasant vacation—because of the organization required beforehand, then the mental awareness needed to navigate unfamiliar territory. If you're traveling for business, most of your focus is directed toward doing well in stressful meetings. A tight schedule doesn't allow much extra time to find a workout facility for physical activity.

Third, if you're traveling with children, ushering them through airports and keeping them happy on long car rides multiplies your stress level severalfold.

So unless you're an athlete with specific goals, or unless you're traveling alone and can wake up for an early morning workout, it's hard to go out and do your physical activity.

As a result, I don't believe you should try any new types of conditioning while you're traveling. You certainly shouldn't seek out the hotel gym to lift weights or figure out how to work the treadmill. Does that surprise you?

It takes months of consistency and progression to achieve any benefits from a new workout. You won't make any new gains by starting a new activity while on the road. Other problems from starting a new routine while traveling include the following:

- ▶ You could get injured. That would certainly take the fun out of your trip.
- ▶ You don't know the quality of the equipment in the gym. Hotel workout equipment is often inferior—if it's not broken.
- ▶ In most cases, there is no staff available to teach you how to use the machines properly and to supervise as you use them.

But in order to maintain the base level of conditioning that you've gained at home—and the improved physical functioning—you can't take off even a few days from your physical activities. Within 24 hours, your neuromuscular system begins to weaken.

So I've devised a simple program that maintains the gains you've made from your *Four Way Burn* activities at home. It consists of a special stretching program and a selection from the 40 techniques you learned earlier. These activities require only a few minutes a day, and you can do them in the comfort of your hotel room. You don't need any special equipment other than your empty carry-on suitcase or a pillow from your bed in place of your ball. You can even do them without holding anything.

SIMPLE STRETCHES KEEP YOU LIMBER

Sitting in a car or an airplane seat for hours at a time makes your muscles stiff and fatigued. That's no way to start a fun vacation or productive business trip. You'll feel better and have more energy by spending just 10 minutes with the following stretching program. (You can call it the "Seated, No-Sweat, Total Body Stretching Program.") The improved flow of oxygen-rich blood throughout your body will reduce stiffness, tightness, and tension, and it will help you feel relaxed.

As soon as you have reached your destination, do a session of stretching. Don't bother changing into exercise clothing. Just pull out a straight-backed chair—most hotel rooms have one—and take a seat.

To get into the starting position, sit upright; don't lean back against the chair back for support. Think tall! Look ahead, without tilting your head forward. Pull your shoulders back and down, and let your arms hang down at your sides. Breathe deeply and rhythmically.

Move through the following steps to relax and stretch your neck and shoulders, back, and lower body.

Neck, shoulders, and upper body

1. Inhale deeply through your nose, and feel your rib cage and chest expanding. Breathe out through your mouth and pull your belly button inward. Repeat three times.

2. Look straight ahead and tilt your head backward. Exhale when you move your head backward, then tilt it forward as you inhale. Keep your eyes forward the entire time and don't move your body. Repeat three times.

3. Interlock your fingers behind your head and tilt your head back again, applying a little force against your head as you press it backward. This strengthens and reinforces your neck muscles to maintain good head alignment. Breathe the same way as above. Repeat three times.

4. Pressing your head to the side against some resistance will strengthen different neck muscles. Place your hand against your temple. Inhale deeply as you push your head toward your shoulder while pushing against the palm of your hand. Repeat on the other side and alternate, three times each side.

5. Turn your head back and forth so that you look over each shoulder. Turn only your head, not your body. Breathe in toward one side and out toward the other side. Repeat three times per side.

6. Roll your head in a half-circle from side to side while you look forward. Move only your head—not your torso. On each side, try to place your ear in line with your shoulder. Inhale as you move your head in both directions. Roll three times in each direction.

7. Reach over your head and interlock your fingers so that the palms of your hands are pointed toward the ceiling. Extend your arms fully upward and feel the stretch in your wrists. Inhale and exhale deeply three times.

8. Interlock your fingers behind your lower back with your palms facing your back. Try to extend your arms behind you and lean forward. Keep your feet firmly on the floor and squeeze your shoulder blades together and downward. You should feel the stretch

in your chest, shoulders, and arms. Breathe in through your nose and out of your mouth three times.

9. Facing forward and sitting upright, hold your arms out to the sides with your palms forward. Breathe out while raising your arms to a hands-up position (as if someone were telling you to "stick 'em up.") Repeat three times.

10. Keep your arms fully extended at your sides. Clench your fists tightly with your thumbs extended. Twist your arms so that your thumbs point behind you. Breathe out while doing so. Repeat three times.

11. Place your hands behind your head and interlock your fingers. Your elbows should point out to your sides. Pull your elbows back three times while breathing out. Feel the stretch in your chest and shoulders as your shoulder blades are pressed together.

12. Lower your arms to your sides and rhythmically roll your shoulders back. Inhale at the lift and exhale as you roll them back three times.

13. Reach over your head with one arm, bend your hand back so that your elbow is pointing up, and place your fingers against the back of your neck. Reach farther down your spine with your fingertips. Assist this stretch by pushing down on your elbow with the opposite hand. Keep your abdominal muscles firm and breathe out each time you reach farther down your neck. Repeat three times. Change arms and repeat.

14. Keep your elbow behind your head and pointed in the air, with your hand hanging down your upper back. Place your other hand against your lower back. Try to reach up your spine with this hand, and reach down with the other to make one concerted effort to close the gap between the fingers on both hands. Breathe out while you're doing this, and don't lean forward. Switch your arm positions and repeat until you've done it three times in each position.

15. Extend both arms out to your sides at shoulder height. Twist your arms in both directions as far as possible. Inhale as you twist toward one direction and exhale as you twist to the other. Keep both elbows in a soft lock. Repeat three times.

Back, hips, and thighs

1. Squeeze your thighs together. With the help of your arms, twist your upper body toward one side and look over your shoulder. While doing so, breathe out. Feel the twist around your waist. Repeat three times in each direction.

2. Return to your starting position. Extend an arm above your head and lean sideways. Bend to the side at your waist and reach out with your hand as far as you can. As you're doing this, keep your legs apart and your feet flat on the floor so that you feel

stable. Keep your head aligned with your spine, and breathe out while reaching. Repeat three times, then repeat on the other side.

3. Place a foot and ankle on top of the opposite thigh. Either hold the foot so that it does not slide down or let your arms hang to your sides. Bend forward from the waist. Feel this stretch in and around your hips, thighs, and lower back. Take three deep breaths, then switch legs and repeat. Maintain a balanced position and keep one foot anchored to the floor throughout the movement.

4. Place both feet flat on the floor and lean forward to touch your toes. Breathe out and suck in your belly button as you bend over. Breathe in as you come up. Repeat three times.

5. Sit in the chair in a neutral position and spread your feet far apart, with your toes pointed outward. Lean forward toward your right foot and reach for your right foot with your left hand. Keep your buttocks completely on the chair. Come back up and repeat on the other side. Alternate sides three times.

6. Lean backward and arch your back. Your arms should be relaxed and hanging at your sides, with the palms of your hands facing forward and your thumbs out. Feel the stretch in your back and the backs of your shoulders. Hold the position for three deep breaths.

7. Hold on to your hips firmly with both hands. Roll your hips forward and back—as in the "suck and tuck" motion—while keeping your upper body stationary. Breathe in as you move toward one direction and breathe out as you move toward the other. Keep your abdominal muscles tight. Repeat three times.

8. Keep your feet flat on the floor and slide them close to the chair. Lean forward slightly from your hips while keeping your back straight. Inhale. Now, stand up straight as you breathe out forcefully. Take another breath and, while breathing out, sit down again. Just touch the chair with your buttocks, then stand back up. Repeat three times.

9. Sit back down. Pull your knee to your chest with your hands as you simultaneously breathe out. Feel your upper and middle back muscles contracting. Switch legs. Repeat three times with each leg.

10. While maintaining a balanced, seated position, shift your weight from one hip to the other. You want to end up sitting momentarily on one buttock, then the other. Breathe out each time you lean. Maintain a balanced and upright position, and keep your feet anchored to the floor at all times. Repeat three times in each direction.

11. Rock your feet forward and back from the heels to the big toes. Inhale deeply toward one direction and exhale toward the other. Repeat three times.

12. Lift one leg off the floor and fully extend it. Breathe out with force as you extend it. Do it with control—not a jerking motion. Repeat three times, then switch to the other leg. Keep the supporting foot anchored to the floor.

13. Turn your entire body toward the right and let only your right hip and buttock rest on the chair. Hold on to the chair for stability. Lunge your left leg back behind your body until you feel a stretch in the front of your left thigh. Take three deep breaths and change sides.

14. Move back to a neutral seated position. To release your body's tension and tightness, squeeze your fists, flex your arms, tighten your jaw, and tighten your thigh and buttock muscles while inhaling. Then exhale and relax all the body parts. Repeat three times.

15. Face forward in a neutral position, with both feet on the floor. Keep your arms at your sides and think peaceful, relaxing thoughts. Breathe in and out of your nose three times.

ADAPT YOUR *FOUR WAY BURN* PROGRAM FOR THE ROAD

The following program is an abbreviated version of the *Four Way Burn* program you do at home. I've chosen 10 techniques that will preserve your strength and flexibility while you're away from home, but that don't require the weighted ball or much space. Instead, use a small object such as a small couch cushion, a pillow off your bed folded in two, a rolled-up bath towel, or your suitcase, if it's relatively small.

Do these in your hotel room every other day. If you have enough space to lie on the floor in a spread-eagle position, you'll have enough room for these techniques.

Do a set of techniques 1 to 3, then do a second set of them. Move on to one set of techniques 4 to 7, then another set. Finish with a set of techniques 8 to 10, then another set.

Good Morning with Side Twist

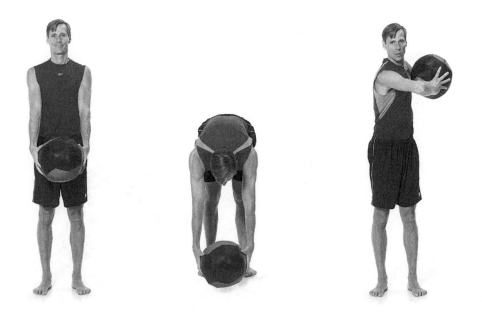

Begin with your feet parallel and closer than shoulder-width apart. At the starting position, hold the ball downward in front of your groin with your arms fully extended.

Lean straight down and touch the ball to the floor in front of your feet. Now, stand up while bringing the ball to your chest, and fully twist your torso to one side. While twisting, make sure that your elbows don't drop below chest level. Return your torso so that you're facing center to complete the repetition. Alternate between twisting left and right with each repetition.

Exhale as you bend down and as you twist.

Straddle Squat and Reach

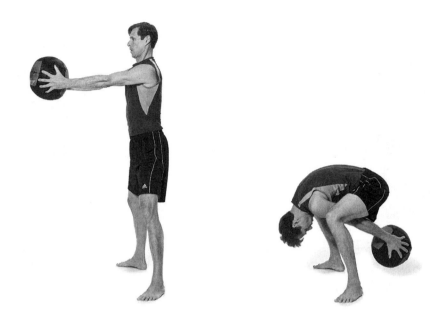

Begin with your feet parallel, but spaced very far apart. Your toes should be pointed outward. Press your big toes into the floor. Hold the ball at arm's length in front of your chest with both hands. Squat down, lean forward, and push the ball between your legs as far back as possible. This time, allow your entire back to become rounded as you push the ball so that you feel a good stretch in your lower back.

Exhale as you reach down, again as you hold the final position, and again as you stand up. Return to the starting point to finish the repetition.

Twist and Sweep

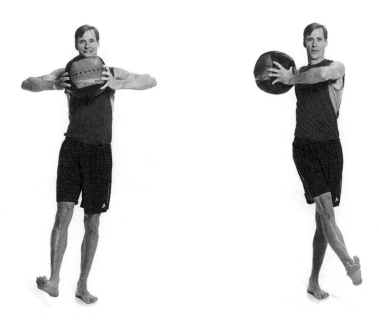

Start by standing on your left foot, with your right foot lifted a few inches in front of you. Hold the ball in front of your chest, with your elbows pointing outward. Twist your upper chest (and the ball) to the right while sweeping your right foot to the left. Your pelvis should stay stationary and your abdominals and lower back should control the motion—but only your chest and leg should move.

During this motion, your standing leg should remain straight and your foot should stay pointing forward. Imagine putting a golf ball with your instep, then with the outer edge of your foot, as your foot sweeps from side to side. Breathe out as you twist in either direction. Complete all repetitions on one side, then switch sides.

Front-Arm Raise with Leg Abduction

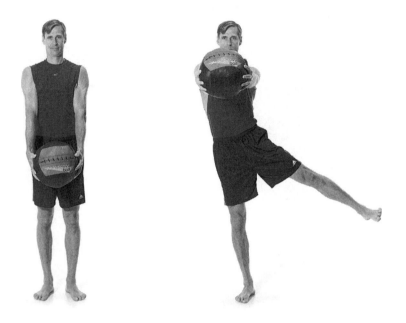

Stand in a parallel stance with your feet shoulder-width apart. Hold the ball in both hands with a strong grip and your arms fully extended, so that the ball is in front of your groin. Lift one leg out to the side while lifting the ball upward until your arms are parallel to the floor, keeping your arms and legs fully extended. To complete the repetition, lower your arms to the starting position and lower your foot until your heels touch. Complete all repetitions, then switch sides and repeat.

Exhale when lifting the ball and again when lowering it.

Adapting *Four Way Burn* for Your Needs

Diagonal Chop

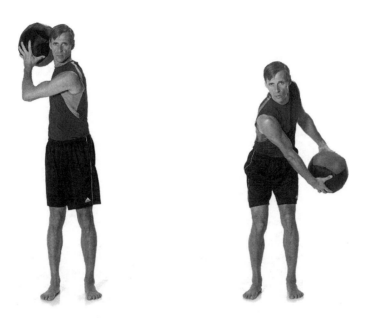

Begin with your feet parallel and less than shoulder-width apart. Hold the ball in both hands over your right shoulder, making sure to not arch your back. Your left shoulder should be relaxed, not shrugged upward, and your torso should be twisted to the right. Maintain a strong grip with both hands.

Move the ball downward toward the floor to your left, taking it on a diagonal path across your body. The ball will end up to the left of your left hip, and your arms will end up straight. Reverse the movement and bring the ball back over your right shoulder to complete the repetition.

Complete all repetitions on one side, then switch sides and repeat. To do the move with the other side of your body, simply start with the ball over your left shoulder and end with it to the right of your right hip.

Breathe out while you're "chopping" the ball down and bringing it up.

Way Down and Way Up

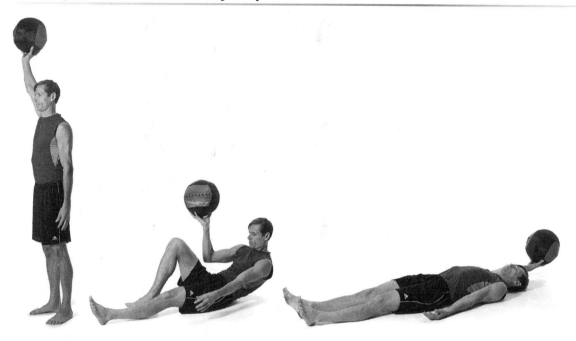

Stand in a parallel stance with your feet a few inches apart, holding the ball in one hand over your head. Slowly lower the ball in front of you, allowing your arm to bend, and lower your buttocks toward the floor. Sit down and lean back, holding the ball aloft. Lie on your back and extend the ball over your head until your arm is parallel with the floor. Slowly raise the ball, sit up, shift your weight, and stand up. Return to the starting position to complete the repetition, switching hands after each repetition. Exhale four times as you go down, and four times as you lift yourself up.

Golfer Swing

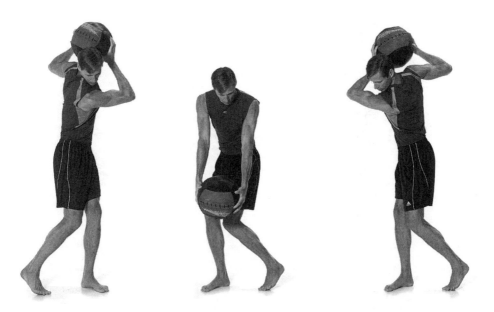

Begin with your feet parallel and less than shoulder-width apart. Extend your arms and hold the ball in front of your groin. Bring the ball up to one shoulder with both hands, as if you're setting up to swing a golf club. Just before you make this motion, start pivoting your feet so that they point toward the direction in which the ball is traveling. Your entire body will be pivoting as you bring the ball above your shoulder. At the highest point, bend both elbows.

When you reach your highest point and have finished the upward motion, pivot your feet the other way and move the ball back down, across your groin and up to your other shoulder. Your arms and the ball will look like a pendulum swinging down and up from shoulder to shoulder as your feet pivot back and forth. Exhale forcefully with each swing. Complete all the repetitions on one side, then switch sides and repeat.

Soldier Walk

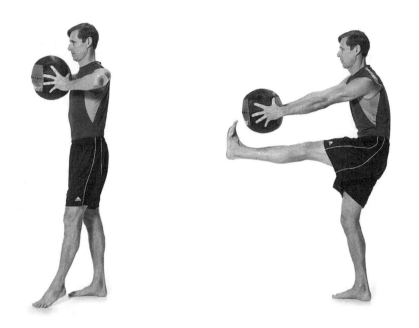

Begin with most of your weight on one foot and the other lightly touching the floor in front of you. Grip the ball in front of your chest with your elbows pointed outward. Lift your front leg while keeping it fully extended. At the same time, push the ball straight out and touch it to your lower shin when your leg reaches its maximum height. Exhale as you touch the ball to your shin.

Keeping your leg fully straightened, lower your foot back to the floor while you pull the ball back to your chest. Complete all repetitions on one side, then switch sides and repeat.

Adapting *Four Way Burn* for Your Needs

Rocking Chair

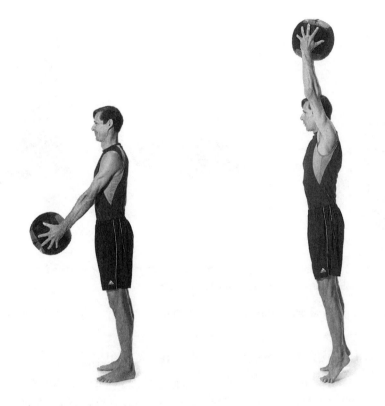

Begin with your feet in a parallel stance, spaced less than shoulder-width apart. Stand up straight and hold the ball so that it's hanging down in front of your groin with your arms fully extended.

Rise up on your toes as you bring the ball straight overhead. Your arms should remain fully extended—never bent—at all times. If you can't bring the ball straight overhead, go as high as your flexibility allows. Now lower the ball back to the starting position as you rock back onto your heels.

Breathe out as you rock back and forth on your feet.

Around the World

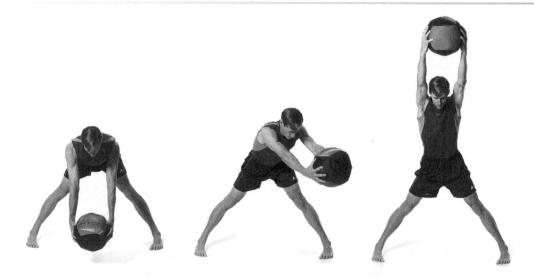

Begin with your feet in a parallel stance, spaced farther than shoulder-width apart. Keep your legs straight, with your toes pointed inward and pressed into the floor.

Lean forward deeply and hold the ball toward the floor in both hands, with your arms fully extended.

Maintain Your Aerobic Routines While Traveling

If you want to keep up your aerobic activities, such as jogging, in addition to your *Four Way Burn* techniques while traveling, it's a good idea to start off slowly until you can adjust to your new surroundings.

I tell people to work out according to either their perceived exertion or their target heart rate.

On a perceived exertion scale, zero is virtually no exertion, 0.5 to 1 is very weak, 1.5 to 2 is weak, 2.5 to 3 is moderate, 4 to 5 is strong, 6 to 7 is very strong, and 8 to 10 is extremely strong.

If you want to exercise according to your target heart rate, first subtract your age from 220. This is your maximum heart rate. If you want to exercise at 50 to 60 percent of your maximum, you'd multiply your maximum by 0.5 and 0.6 to find the range. For a 40-year-old, the maximum would be 180, and 50 to 60 percent of the maximum would be 90 to 108 beats per minute.

On the first day of travel, do your aerobic activities at only a 5 to 6 on the exertion scale, or at 50 to 60 percent of your maximum heart rate.

Over the next few days, slowly build up to the level of exertion that you use at home, not exceeding 80 percent of your maximum heart rate unless recommended by your doctor.

Adapting *Four Way Burn* for Your Needs

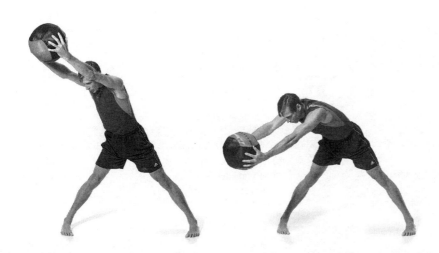

Reaching out as far as you can, move the ball out to your left and up until it's overhead, then on to your right, and back down to the starting point. As you reach the high point of this circle, stretch yourself up as tall as you can. Keep your arms and legs straight as you make the circle. Finish all the repetitions in one direction, then switch directions.

Exhale as your hands travel past each quarter of the circle.

TRAVELERS' PROGRAM CHART

Good Morning with Side Twist	5 reps for beginner, each side 8 reps for intermediate 10 reps for advanced
Straddle Squat and Reach	5 reps for beginner 10 reps for intermediate 15 reps for advanced
Twist and Sweep	5 reps for beginner 8 reps for intermediate 10 reps for advanced

Do a second set of the first three techniques, then move on to the next group.

Front-Arm Raise with Leg Abduction	10 reps for beginner 15 reps for intermediate 20 reps for advanced
Diagonal Chop	10 reps for beginner 15 reps for intermediate 20 reps for advanced
Way Down and Way Up	10 reps for beginner 15 reps for intermediate 20 reps for advanced
Golfer Swing	10 reps for beginner 15 reps for intermediate 20 reps for advanced

Do a second set of the second four techniques, then move on to the last group.

Soldier Walk	10 reps for beginner 15 reps for intermediate 20 reps for advanced
Rocking Chair	10 reps for beginner 15 reps for intermediate 20 reps for advanced
Around the World	10 reps for beginner 15 reps for intermediate 20 reps for advanced

Do a second set of the last group of three techniques.

8

LOSE WEIGHT WITH
FOUR WAY BURN

Sometimes, it seems like nearly everyone on the planet would like to exercise more, eat a healthier diet, and lose weight. However, most people never actually accomplish these goals for any significant length of time.

That's because many people pin their hopes on magic formulas for quick weight loss—but there are none. They may take a few steps toward their goal, but after they have a bad day or two, they go back to their usual habits. Their weight continues to increase, and eventually, it affects their health.

The keys to weight loss aren't magic, but they are simple: For starters, you must eat and drink fewer calories than you use for metabolism and physical activity. Or, if you want to look at it another way, you have to use more calories than you consume. The number of calories you use each day depends in large part on how physically active you are and how much muscle mass you have in your body.

To use more calories, you need to move around every day. Some people call this exercise, but I don't like that word—it makes moving sound like a chore. I prefer the term *physical activity.* Your body was made to move. It *wants* to move. Movement keeps it healthy.

Unfortunately, as seen with our skyrocketing healthcare costs, we're defying these basic principles. Many people keep indulging themselves with more calories from food and beverages than they're burning off through physical activity.

Food and beverage advertisements on television, radio, magazines, and websites reinforce a culture in which we're accustomed to supersizing our cheeseburgers and sodas. And we are buying lots of needless food—it is just too hard to resist.

In addition, businesses have become more competitive, which means that workers have less time for lunch breaks, and they stay at work later because of deadlines. Take-out food has replaced home cooking. Fast food is filling for the body (and for many people, it's calming for the mind), but it's usually very dense in calories.

I can't stress it enough: In order to live a healthier and happier life, you must learn to eat less and become more active. But this doesn't mean that you have to starve yourself and spend 10 hours a day doing situps. If you want to lose weight and keep it off, it is important to make small, gradual changes so that you shed your weight gradually over a period of time.

You probably know people who have lost a lot of weight quickly, perhaps to get in shape before a vacation or a class reunion. But in most of these cases, the weight will quickly return. Statistics show that most people who lose a significant amount of weight (3 pounds or more per week) will have a difficult time sustaining the discipline they need to maintain their weight loss.

The healthiest way to lose weight, which offers the best chance of long-term success, is to start by aiming to lose 10 percent of your current body weight over 6 months. Plan to lose no more than a pound or two a week so that you can lose weight in the form of fat, and not just water—which is a temporary loss—or muscle, which you want to maintain.

Want Weight Loss? Do the Math

One pound of fat equals 3,500 calories. If you consume 3,500 more calories than you burn off through physical activity, you gain a pound. If you burn off 3,500 more than you consume, you lose a pound. To lose 2 pounds a week means you need to run a deficit of 7,000 calories through more activity and less consumption each week. That means burning 500 more calories a day and eating 500 fewer calories a day.

Most people consume 2,500 to 3,500—or more—calories per day. However, a nutritious, balanced diet containing about 1,500 to 1,800 calories for women or 1,800 to 2,200 calories for men is enough to allow people to take in all the vitamins and minerals they need to support a healthy and functional body and mind while they lose weight. Also, when you're losing weight, you may not eat enough from all of the food groups each day, so taking a multivitamin and mineral tablet is a good idea.

THE DIET COMPONENT OF WEIGHT LOSS: MAKE MANY SMALL CHANGES

We are creatures of habit, and companies that market fattening foods rely on our predictable nature to make lots of sales. You buy large portions of unhealthy foods at supermarkets and restaurants because you have come to think that's just the normal way to eat.

It's time to start becoming wary of the type of lifestyle you see advertised. The reality is that you have to be in control of your life in order to lose weight and keep it off. You have to be accountable for your actions.

Below, I will suggest ways to modify your eating habits so you can lose weight. Making these small changes will help change your diet to encourage permanent weight loss. But don't use these as your only changes. Once you have read this chapter, you might come up with your own helpful steps that meet your specific needs and lifestyle.

The main food-related change you need to make is to simply eat less . . . and *not* to change the types of foods you eat. I don't think people who want to lose weight should be focused on eating fewer carbs or less fat or more protein or more bowls of cabbage soup. You've spent many years feeding your body the same sorts of foods, and it's grown accustomed to that.

To lose weight, you need to eat fewer calories and expend more calories through physical activity. Overhauling your menu on top of these other lifestyle improvements requires your body to adjust to too many changes at one time. So I'm not going to tell you to change the amount of fat, carbs, or protein that you eat. I'm not going to give you a list of good and bad foods, either.

I just want you, at least for right now, to cut back on the portions you eat. Make lots of little changes to your eating habits to help you eat less. Your body can get used to this new "setpoint" when you feed it fewer calories slowly and gradually. Your mind won't get as antsy as it does when you're suddenly not eating the foods to which you're accustomed.

Most people stay in the phase in which they just *contemplate* making lasting changes. They just keep thinking about it. We need to get to the execution phase. Don't just think about it—*do* it! Start making these little changes one at a time.

The first week will be the hardest for resisting the temptation to quit. Be tough, and override your old habits. Find alternatives to occupy yourself without eating. Pick up a book you haven't read, or do tasks around the house that you've meant to do for some time but have put off. Keep yourself busy, and before you know it, something wonderful will have happened.

Your stomach will shrink and the urge for more food will calm down. Because the changes are small, you won't really notice any major difference in your life. Your mind won't rebel against your new lifestyle and start providing reasons why you should give up on your weight-loss plan.

General food guidelines

To reduce your calorie consumption, follow these suggestions:

▶ Do not change your usual food choices, at least at first. Focus instead on taking smaller portions.

Weight-Loss Portraits of Success

What has kept you from losing weight and keeping it off in the past? Do you find physical activity too tiring or boring? Do you lack the willpower to make permanent changes to your diet?

I've worked with a lot of people who faced significant challenges that could have kept them from losing weight. They had injuries. They had little time. They loved their food. But they succeeded.

The people I know who have kept the weight off share some common traits:

▶ They can find pleasure in other things besides eating and drinking—in particular, moving their bodies.

▶ They understand that they won't live forever, and they want to make the most of the time they have been given.

▶ They can remain organized and stick with a structure.

▶ They can say "no thank you" to food and "yes, I can and I will" to physical activity.

Here's a quick look at some of my clients' success stories. Their names are changed, but their stories are very true.

Robert. Shortly after he started training, he discovered a herniated disk in his back, and his physician suggested surgery. I convinced him to stay put and strengthen his abdominals and back muscles. With some integrated stretches, he quickly felt better, and he never went under the knife. Twice a week he gets his "Ralf" sessions, but he also works out four or five times per week on his own at home. He has kept his weight constant through hard times in his life, and he knows how important it is to *not* stop moving his body.

Nora. She was relatively healthy and active, but she joined one of my fitness classes

- ▶ Eat your regular breakfast.
- ▶ Eat one-quarter less lunch. Reduce an even amount of food from all the food groups— don't just cut out lots of your veggies. Walk around the block or up the stairs with the few minutes you save by not eating as much.
- ▶ Before lunch and dinner, drink two glasses of water. This will help fill you up.
- ▶ Eat one-third less dinner. Again, spend the minutes you save moving your body around a little.

because she wanted to add a fun and social element to exercising. She also wanted to practice functional skills such as balance, coordination, and agility in her physical activity regimen. Ever since we met 10 years ago, she's been training with me, and she remains in good enough shape to play tennis and ski with her adolescent sons.

Frank. Even though he runs a global business, Frank finds time to train with me almost daily. Since he began working with me, his muscle mass has increased, his body fat has decreased, and he has resolved his knee, back, and shoulder problems. His challenging program featuring the Performance Ball, a balance beam, and a trampoline enhances his control over his body while it's in motion. This has improved his tennis, skiing, and mountain biking.

Tom. He was wheelchair-bound when we met, after being injured by a delivery truck that hit him broadside. His regimen was nothing more than a specially designed strength and conditioning program for his specific needs. Over time, with a lot of hard work, he became a fully independent person who plays golf, lives on his own, and *doesn't* need a wheelchair.

Ben. He came to me weighing too much, stuck in a sedentary lifestyle, and suffering from diabetes. Ben's schedule as a writer left no time for physical activity, but he needed to change his lifestyle by controlling his diet and beginning a structured cardiovascular program. He began walking 30 minutes daily and cut down on meat and dairy products to reduce his calorie intake by one-third. After just 3 months, his doctor took him off the cholesterol medication he had prescribed earlier.

John. When he started working with me, John had a 52-inch waistline. We designed a program of daily walking or another form of aerobic activity along with strength-training activities to boost his metabolism and to keep his joints strong. After 2 years of his new lifestyle, he had lost 100 pounds and trimmed down to a 34-inch waist. He has kept this weight off for the last 10 years.

- Eat your final meal by 7:00 p.m. Once you finish dinner, stop eating for the day.

- Do some physical activities after dinner.

- Reduce your alcohol consumption by 50 percent. Better yet, cut it out entirely. Alcohol invites excess eating.

- Replace all your plates, bowls, cups, and other dishes with smaller ones.

- Reduce your soda consumption by 50 percent, or cut it out entirely.

- Cut back on desserts by 75 percent. Or cut them out entirely. Why do you really need a dessert? You just finished eating an entire meal! You can lose 10 pounds per year just by not eating dessert regularly.

- Skip your coffee break in the afternoon. Go for a walk instead.

- Look for places to trim out a few calories—they can really add up. For example, just by changing from cream to fat-free milk in your coffee, you can lose 7 to 10 pounds a year.

- If you come home from work hungry, drink water and eat a high-fiber snack before dinner, such as carrots. It will fill you up.

- Leave the skin on fruits and vegetables. It helps fill you up without adding extra calories. This roughage also helps clean out your digestive tract as the food passes through your system.

- Remove the skin—and the underlying layer of fat—from chicken, turkey, and other poultry before you cook it. To replace the moisture and flavor, marinate the meat before cooking.

- Eat an extra-large portion of salad before your dinner. It will help fill you up before you eat higher-calorie foods.

- When you're watching television, skip the commercials. Every other commercial is about food and drinks, anyway. Do some housework for a few minutes instead, such as folding laundry, clearing dishes, or cleaning. Or avoid TV entirely, and read more.

- Dilute any juice by 50 percent with tap water or sparkling water.

- Drink fat-free milk instead of whole milk.

- It's okay to go to bed a little hungry. You won't wake up hungry, because while you are sleeping, your body snacks on its stored fat. While you sleep, you actually burn a decent number of calories.

- Wash and dry your dishes by hand instead of using the dishwasher. Let the children help. It's social, it's fun, and it burns calories.

- Always have healthy snacks available, such as carrots, cherry tomatoes, and pretzels.

- Find pleasure in activities other than eating and drinking.

Healthful food shopping

By using a shopping list and keeping your kitchen well stocked with nutritious foods, you can reduce the time required to prepare healthy meals. Read the labels as you shop, and pay attention to serving size and servings per container. Compare the total calories in similar products and choose the one with fewer calories.

Here's how to come away from the store with foods that will help you lose weight:

- ▶ Have a food budget and stick with it. This will leave less money to buy junk food and snacks, and it will save you money for your next active vacation.
- ▶ Load up on lots of veggies and fruits first. Then go for complex carbohydrates such as whole grains. Then buy a smaller amount of meat and other animal foods. At the end, buy frozen processed meals, ice cream, and candy very sparingly.
- ▶ Don't even go down the aisle where sodas and chips are located. You can resist them!
- ▶ Eat more fresh fish, such as tuna, salmon, and flounder.
- ▶ When you buy meat, choose leaner cuts, such as pork loin instead of pork ribs, and chicken breast instead of chicken thighs.
- ▶ When buying cold cuts at the deli, ask for them to be sliced extra-thin. You can serve yourself a smaller portion of thinly sliced meats.
- ▶ When you make a sandwich, use small-size pieces of bread. Instead of fatty mayonnaise, use low-calorie condiments such as ketchup, mustard, and pickles.
- ▶ Most dairy products, such as cheese and yogurt, come in lower-calorie versions. Buy those.
- ▶ Stay organized while you're shopping. Don't stray. Stick to the list you made before you arrived at the store.
- ▶ Make your shopping time an organized physical activity. Keep moving and stop only to load your cart.

Remember: If you don't have it at home, you won't consume it. So don't stock up on foods and beverages that are low in nutritional value. The temptation to eat them once you bring them home is too large.

Eating right at restaurants

It's easy to fill up on fatty, high-calorie foods when you're eating in restaurants. Owners of restaurants want you to keep coming back, so they serve you tasty foods in big portions. Believe me—as a former chef and restaurant owner, I know.

Load Up on These Weight-Loss Foods

Make room in your shopping cart for these lower-calorie items that make great components of nutritious meals:

- Fat-free or low-fat milk, yogurt, cheese, and cottage cheese
- Light margarine
- Eggs or egg substitutes
- Whole wheat sandwich breads, bagels, pita, and English muffins
- Soft corn tortillas or low-fat flour tortillas
- Low-fat, low-sodium crackers
- Plain cereal, dry or cooked
- Whole grain rice
- Whole wheat pasta
- White meat chicken or turkey (remove the skin)

- Fish and shellfish (not battered)
- Beef: round, sirloin, chuck arm, loin, and extra-lean ground beef
- Pork: leg, shoulder, tenderloin
- Dry beans and peas
- Fresh, frozen, or canned fruits in light syrup or juice
- Fresh, frozen, or no-salt-added canned vegetables
- Low-fat or fat-free salad dressings
- Mustard and ketchup
- Jam, jelly, or honey
- Herbs and spices

But I also know that restaurants offer the foods that people want, and many people are interested in more nutritious menu items nowadays. You can make some simple choices when you're eating out so that you can enjoy great foods while limiting your calorie consumption:

- Make your reservations for early in the evening. If you wait too late to eat, you become hungry and you overeat once you take a place at the table.
- Order water or sparkling water before the meal to help fill your stomach.
- Decline the bread basket before the meal, and ask the waiter to remove the butter from your table.
- If you must drink alcohol, order no more than half a bottle of wine, or order by the glass. Put ice cubes in your wine glass to "stretch" the wine. Try it—it really works!
- Also, if you must drink, have a cocktail or wine—not both.

Adapting *Four Way Burn* for Your Needs

- ▶ Order a healthful appetizer as your main course.
- ▶ Opt for a broth instead of a cream-based soup.
- ▶ Ask what low-calorie dishes are available on the menu.
- ▶ Ask for your entrée to be broiled or boiled instead of fried or sautéed.
- ▶ Stay busy talking, and eat less. Make it a social event.
- ▶ Have coffee or tea afterward, but skip the dessert. Or split one dessert into smaller portions and share.
- ▶ Take a walk after the meal.

TO BURN CALORIES, KEEP YOUR BODY MOVING

The *Four Way Burn* program gives you many types of physical improvement in one session. You become more flexible by stretching your muscles. Your heart and lungs get a similar workout as they would with swimming, jogging, or other aerobic activities. And because you're lifting a 4- to 6-pound weight countless times in many directions, you get a great strength-training session.

However, I intend for you to use my program only 3 days a week. That means that you should perform other physical activities on another 3 days each week. This is particularly important if your goal is to lose weight.

Ideally, you should accumulate at least an hour of physical activity each day. If you don't have an entire hour to devote to it at one time, break it up into smaller segments. Remember: The benefits of physical activity accumulate, just as your weight accumulated over time.

The more your entire body is engaged in moving, the more calories you'll burn. Also, the harder you perceive your effort to be during a given activity, the more calories you'll burn. Try to move extra-vigorously during at least half an hour of your physical activity so that you can burn more calories. An easy way to know whether you're working vigorously is that the exertion will make you breathe heavily.

For examples of physical activities that will strengthen your heart and lungs—and burn lots of calories—check out the options on page 114. Many of these are fun. Others aren't necessarily fun, but they *will* make your home cleaner. Keep in mind that some sports, such as baseball or softball, include a lot of downtime, and it's difficult to tell how much time you're actually moving. Focus more on activities that involve continuous movement.

Keep Trying New Physical Activities

Time constraints, lack of energy, lack of interest, and other reasons can make it difficult for many people to get the daily physical activity they need to lose 2 pounds a week. To keep your physical activities fun and challenging, try two or more of the options from this list each week, in addition to your *Four Way Burn* sessions.

▶ Basketball

▶ Soccer

▶ Volleyball and beach volleyball

▶ Walking over hills

▶ Running

▶ Dancing

▶ Racquetball

▶ Tennis

▶ Squash

▶ Rock climbing

▶ Boxing, kickboxing, karate, and other martial arts

▶ Fencing

▶ Cycling (indoors or outdoors) and mountain biking

▶ Jumping rope

▶ Rowing

▶ Ice skating and speed skating

▶ Hockey

▶ Trampoline jumping

▶ Swimming

▶ Skiing (cross-country or downhill)

▶ Waterskiing

▶ Snowboarding

▶ Sledding

▶ Stairclimbing machines

▶ Weight training

▶ Playing actively with your children

Many chores and household tasks will also count toward your hour of daily physical activity, including:

▶ Cleaning floors

▶ Raking leaves

▶ Shoveling snow

▶ Vacuuming

▶ Painting

▶ Pruning trees

▶ Loading and unloading groceries

▶ Moving furniture

▶ Washing the car

▶ Climbing stairs

▶ Making the bed

And keep in mind the pillars of my philosophy on health and fitness:

▶ We are required to move for a healthy mind and strong bones, joints, and muscles.

▶ We must move daily.

▶ We must move *all* of our body parts and muscle groups to prevent atrophy and deterioration.

▶ No matter what the weather—hot or cold—get outside and move around. Enjoy the world around you. Seeing, smelling, and feeling the world lets you know that you're alive.

▶ The phrase "If you don't use it, you will lose it" is very true.

▶ We can sit and rest, but only after we have moved.

▶ Moving comes in all forms and shapes. Choose your favorite activities and do them!

Strength training: Don't forget these weight-loss activities

The list of health benefits you get from strength training reads like a visit to the fountain of youth. When you build muscle through strength training—such as the *Four Way Burn* program or lifting weights—the added muscle burns more calories and thus can help you lose weight or maintain your weight loss.

Strength training can improve your mood and relieve depression. It can help increase your balance and kinesthetic awareness, which makes moving around a whole lot easier and helps prevent injury. Being stronger also helps improve your ability to do aerobic activities.

Strength training uses resistance methods to increase your ability to exert or resist a physical force. The resistance you work against could come from free weights, machines, rubber tubing, or just your body weight. The way you build your strength in the *Four Way Burn* program is with a weighted ball.

Strengthening your muscles becomes more important as you progress through adulthood. Research shows that your muscle strength decreases by 15 percent each decade after you turn 50. After the age of 70, it dwindles by 30 percent each decade.

As a result, even if your weight stays the same, over the decades, more of your weight may be from fat and less from muscle, but you may not realize that this change is happening. Women's body fat percentage should remain between 18 and 25 percent, and men's should be between 12 and 18 percent. (To find out your percentage, ask a qualified personal trainer or other fitness professional.)

By doing strength training, you'll help ensure that more of your weight is composed of useful muscle—not needless fat. The decrease in muscle tissue and strength that can occur throughout life isn't a natural result of aging—it's from lack of use!

I'm interested in helping people become more fit so they can look better, but more importantly, I want their bodies to *function* better in everyday life. Strength gains can lead to greater walking speed, more stairclimbing power, and better balance. An increase in strength can make the difference between being able to get up from a chair by yourself someday or having to wait for someone to help you get up. This is true functional improvement.

As you learned from doing the *Four Way Burn* activities earlier in the book, you don't need to own special clothing, barbells, or a membership to a fitness club to do strength training. All you need is a positive attitude and a few spare minutes.

You learned plenty of good reasons throughout this book why my program should remain a vital part of your fitness routine for the rest of your life. Losing extra weight and keeping it off is yet another good reason.

So keep picking up that weighted ball and working through your 40 activities! Your slimmer body will keep thanking you.

The *Four Way Burn* Strength and Conditioning Plus Weight-Loss Program

To incorporate the *Four Way Burn* program into an overall weight-loss plan, do the program 3 days a week, and spend the same amount of time on alternate days doing cardio training. Take the seventh day off.

Why should you spend a similar amount of time on aerobic training and strength training? Maintaining a balance of activities keeps your musculoskeletal system evenly trained with your cardiopulmonary system (your heart and lungs). You'll also help prevent injuries and burnout over the long term.

Here's a sample pace you might want to maintain during each cardio session if you choose to run or bicycle. Just as the *Four Way Burn* program requires you to gradually increase the challenge while doing activities with the weighted ball, the schedule below will also allow you to gradually add new challenges for your body as you become more fit.

	BEGINNER PACE	INTERMEDIATE PACE	ADVANCED PACE
Walkers/runners	3.5 mph	4–6.5 mph	7+ mph
Bicyclists	12 mph	13–17 mph	18+ mph

9

THE RIGHT MOVES CAN BRING BACK YOUR STRONG, FLEXIBLE BACK

America and other industrialized nations keep growing and moving forward because millions of their citizens stay seated. Day after day, many people sit in their office chairs, doing their work with computers and phones.

Previous generations relied on their strong backs to help them work hard. Nowadays, people develop *weakened* backs from working at sedentary jobs. Ironic, isn't it?

According to the National Institutes of Health, "nearly everyone" will have significant back pain at some point in their lives. Lower back pain is the most common source of job-related disability in America, and it costs at least $50 billion a year.

The most common sources of back problems include:

Lack of activity. Back stiffness can result from the sedentary lifestyle that involves too much sitting down at work and at home. The muscles and connective tissue in your back become too weak to support and accommodate moving body parts. Weak muscles, tendons, and ligaments can become injured from even small, basic movements such as picking up a newspaper or taking a shower.

Weak or tight muscles elsewhere in your body can lead to back problems, too. For example, a tight hamstring behind your thigh will cause difficulty in lifting your leg. Because this muscle is in close proximity to your lower back, when it's tight and weak, the muscles nearby will suffer, too.

Stress. The pressure of performing and delivering results at work is higher than ever. If you have a high-pressure job—or other source of stress, for that matter—it can cause muscles in your neck and back to grow tense, which ultimately causes pain.

Weight. Carrying too much weight—an issue for the majority of Americans—is a major factor in back pain, too.

Consider pregnant women: As they gain weight in the front, pregnant women must make adjustments to maintain their center of balance while moving around. They arch their backs more and shift their weight back to their heels while walking. This compresses the vertebrae in the lower back and throws their bodies out of normal alignment.

The same thing can happen to people who simply put on excess weight. Over time—often over decades—people can gain 15 to 20 pounds without noticing it. The body tries to accommodate these gains, but gradually, the resulting shift away from the body's natural balance causes pain.

Often when people's backs become stiff and painful—from stress, from being overweight, or for whatever other reason—they limit their physical activities to protect against further pain. However, that's generally the wrong thing to do. You want to stay active to increase your back's flexibility. The lack of activity from prolonged rest makes it even more stiff and susceptible to injury.

If you often have back pain and stiffness, this chapter is for you. I'll lay out an activity program at the end of the chapter that you should do to strengthen your back and give it flexibility. Once you complete this program and your back feels better, then you can go on to begin the four cycles of the *Four Way Burn* program that make up the central focus of the book.

If you presently have a back injury or pain, talk to your physician before beginning the program in this chapter. It's intended for people with periodic back problems, but not a present acute injury.

First, let's learn a little more about back pain and health.

THE COMPONENTS OF A PAIN-FREE BACK

Imagine a model skeleton hanging in a doctor's office or anatomy classroom. The long, flexible spine holds the weight of the rest of the skeleton as if it were a string supporting all these other parts.

Your own spine is very similar. Your lower back is a potentially weak link in your body since it's a region that has to carry, absorb, and redirect energy from your upper body to your lower body, and vice versa. It plays a crucial role when you carry weight, when you walk, when you bend over, and when you twist your upper body. When you consider that you usually do these movements in various combinations at one time, it's not surprising that your back needs a lot of strength and flexibility to stay healthy.

The key elements for keeping or achieving a healthy back are:

Strong muscles. Many people have the misconception that by doing crunches or situps and strengthening the abdominals, they also strengthen the lower back.

It's true that these movements will stretch the lower back and therefore improve or at least maintain its flexibility. The abdominal muscles also support the lower back while in motion, because they are connected to the lower back via a system of muscles and joints. And strong abdominal muscles—not the outer layers but the deep abdominal layers—strengthen and support the pelvis, which helps align and support the spine above. (The muscles that create the distinctive "six-pack" look offer relatively little support to the lower back.)

However, to strengthen your lower back, you must condition it with other moves besides situps and crunches. Your lower back's role in your body's functioning requires it to lift your body weight—plus any weight you're carrying—while you're twisting and turning. As a result, movements to strengthen your back should require you to lift and lower your body while doing some twisting on the way down and up. This helps integrate your lower back into the rest of the "chain" of interconnected body parts.

Flexibility. You need limber muscles and a good range of motion to protect your lower back. The lower back functions best when its strength and flexibility are balanced out in both directions—also called flexion (when you lean forward) and extension (when you lean back). Conditioning techniques that improve the health of your back need to incorporate these motions, too.

Good posture and body alignment. When you do your daily activities, you must move in a way that's proper for your body. Good form is also important when you play sports so that you don't put needless stress on your frame.

Even if you do put on some extra weight, it doesn't necessarily have to interfere with good body alignment. One can be healthy and relatively fit, even with a few extra pounds. But it is imperative that you balance out your body weight with the right amount of strength and flexibility to support your skeleton while it's in motion. If you neglect your alignment, back problems and other orthopedic problems will occur.

It's easy to work on good balance, posture, and alignment. All you need is a wall. But if you don't have a wall, you can do an alternative technique on a floor. Give these a try.

▶ **The wall technique for improving your posture.** Begin by standing with your back against the wall. Try to place the back of your head and your shoulders, buttocks, and heels against the wall. Suck in your belly button and stand tall. Hold this position for several moments, and practice it often. The more you practice, the more you become aware of good posture and maintain it during the day.

▶ **The floor technique for improving your posture.** Lie on the floor with your arms and legs fully extended, your palms facing the ceiling, and your chin tucked. Simultaneously press the back of your head into the floor and do the "suck and tuck" motion—which means you squeeze your buttocks and suck in your belly button to tilt your pelvis forward. Do these motions rhythmically as you breathe, and repeat 20 times. This gives you a good sense of your body's alignment so you can hold yourself in the proper position during the day.

Proper ergonomics. Your office chair and computer need to be adjustable so that they're at the right height.

Also, here is a tip for keeping your body in the proper position while sitting: Sit with both buttocks evenly on the chair, with your thighs parallel to the floor and both feet planted on the floor. Your head should be erect, your ears should be over your shoulders, and your chin in, your chest out, and your shoulders back and down. Allow your arms to hang relaxed at your sides.

Now, breathe in deeply through your nose and exhale through your mouth. Repeat 10 times while maintaining good posture and proper alignment and focusing on holding your body tall and erect. This may be done several times a day as a refreshing break while you're at the computer or doing paperwork.

Another way to keep your body limber during the day is to do the seated stretches from pages 88 to 92 in Chapter 7. If you sit much of the day at work, do these stretches from time to time to prevent stiffness.

MAKING THE RIGHT MOVES TO RESTORE YOUR BACK

A common misconception is that complete rest is necessary for treating back pain. However, the body is meant to move, not sit still, and in most cases, rest doesn't cure back pain as well as movement does. Plus, if you don't get to the fundamental problem of your lack of strength and flexibility, these painful episodes will return.

A colleague and friend of mine, Evan Karas, MD, an orthopedic surgeon in New York, agrees. "Aerobic exercise has been shown to be extremely beneficial for people with back pain. You just need to be educated on how to exercise properly and get that aerobic exercise without putting stress on the lower back. For example, instead of doing exercises that are weight bearing, try doing less-weight-bearing exercises, like bicycling. Also, swimming takes a lot of stress off the lower back while you get aerobic exercise," he says.

Long-term pain relief is possible! The recipe for curing back pain is often a simple combination of exercise involving strengthening and stretching, combined with proper ergonomics and good posture.

A modified version of the *Four Way Burn* program can gently put your back through a range of motions that improve its strength and mobility. However, it's possible that these conditioning measures will cause a bit of soreness before they bring relief.

Feeling sore is actually an indicator that you have moved out of your comfort zone. The stimulation of your tissues through activity—if not overdone—will ensure that they grow stronger, or at least hold their strength. If you follow my back conditioning program, you will experience some soreness at times, but you shouldn't feel pain.

As you rest between sessions, the tissues that you worked may feel sore as they grow stronger so they can accommodate the next workout. Doing three sessions per week will ensure that you attain growth and proper recovery without overworking yourself.

It is also important to understand that your circulatory system carries accumulated waste away from the areas that have been working, and at the same time it replenishes and brings new nutrients to them for healing and growth.

That's why you need to take it easy on the days between sessions, but still move around. Getting some aerobic activity will help the waste "flush out" faster than if you sit or lie down. So be sure to walk or do other activities on the days between the sessions of the following program.

THE 8-WEEK BACK PROGRAM

The following program consists of four 2-week cycles. Each cycle requires you to do seven sessions, one every other day, so you'll do them Monday, Wednesday, Friday, Sunday, Tuesday, Thursday, and Saturday. Then you'll move to the next cycle.

You can do these at a beginner, intermediate, or advanced level. The only difference between the levels is the number of repetitions.

Seated Side Twist

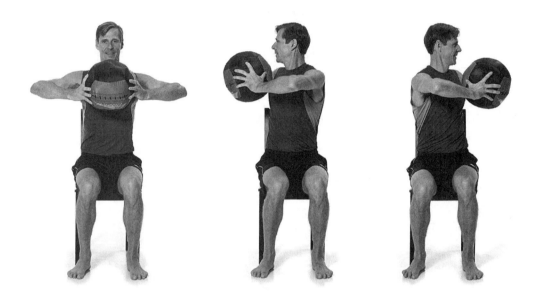

Sit on a firm chair or bench with your feet on the floor in front of you. Hold the ball with both hands in front of your chest, with your elbows pointing out to the sides. Begin twisting your torso from side to side, using the core muscles around your abdomen and lower back to provide movement. Each repetition requires you to fully twist one way, then the other. Exhale one long breath as you move in each direction.

Seated Good Morning

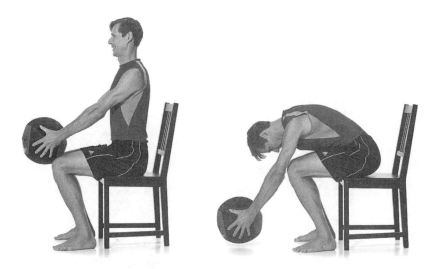

Sit on a firm chair or bench with your feet on the floor in front of you. Bend over at your hips and hold the ball downward with your arms fully extended. Push the ball down to the floor near your feet, or as close to the floor as you can.

Sit back most of the way up, but not completely upright, while keeping your arms fully extended toward the floor. Exhale as you move in each direction.

Wall Squat

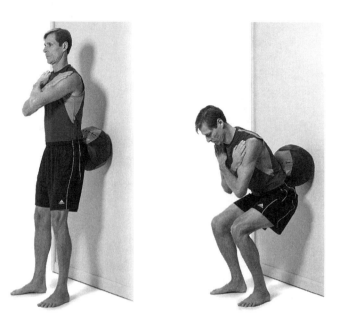

Stand with your back to a wall and ball held between the wall and your lower back and buttocks. Cross your arms over your chest, keep your feet flat on the floor, and squat slightly so that your legs are bent at a 45-degree angle.

Look down. You should not see your toes or feet—they should be hidden behind your knees. Now, lean forward with your upper body as if you were trying to see whether your shoelaces were untied. Hold the position and count slowly to 40. Breathe deeply and rhythmically. You may feel your lower back and thighs getting tired, since this technique strengthens these regions.

Reach, Tuck, and Touch

Kneel down and place your knees and palms on the floor so that you're on all fours. Keep your knees a few inches apart and your hands shoulder-width apart. Lift your left leg off the floor and straighten it fully behind you, parallel with the floor. With your right hand, pick up your ball and lift it. Try to reach far out. You are now balancing yourself on your left hand and your right knee.

Pull your right arm and left leg back toward your center and try to touch your right elbow to your left knee. Re-extend your arm and leg and repeat for the full number of repetitions, then change sides. Breathe out with each reach and with each elbow-to-knee touch.

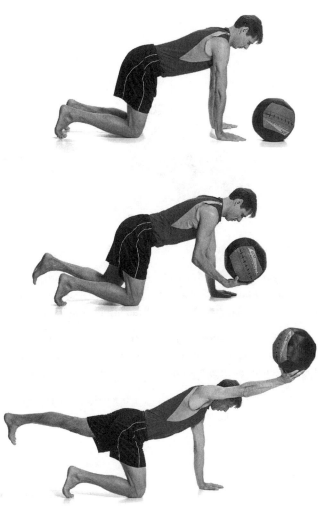

Lying Side Twist

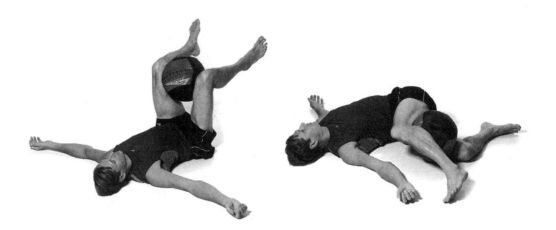

Lie with your back on a firm surface, bend your legs with your feet flat on the floor, and place the ball between your knees and inner thighs. Extend your arms out at chest level, with your palms facing the ceiling. Press your upper back and head firmly down to the floor.

Now, pull your knees toward your chest and lower your legs to the right, rotating at your hips. Your right thigh will end up resting on the floor. Continue to roll your left leg slightly farther over the top of the ball. Now, turn your head to the left, and rotate your knees and the ball over to the left.

Breathe deeply in and out of your nose three times while your legs are lowered to each side. Repeat a second set, if desired.

Side Twist

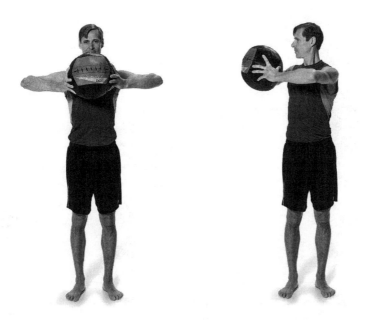

Begin with your feet in a parallel stance, with your hands holding the ball in front of your chest and your elbows pointing out to the sides. Begin twisting your torso from side to side, using the core muscles around your abdomen and lower back to provide movement. You're only twisting your upper body—you're not twisting at the knees. Each repetition requires you to fully twist one way, then the other.

Exhale one long breath as you move in each direction.

Squat and Reach

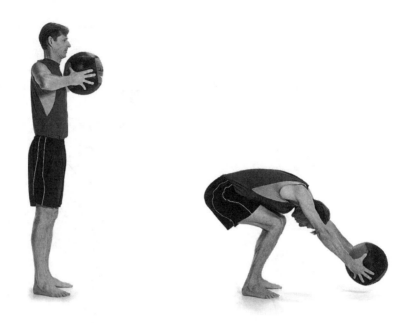

Stand in a parallel stance, holding the ball at your chest with your elbows out. Squat down and extend your arms so that you're reaching out toward the floor away from your feet with the ball. You should feel the stretch in your lower back. Keep your heels on the floor at all times.

Bridging

Lie on your back on the floor, with the ball resting on the floor next to your right hip. Bend your knees and place your feet flat on the floor. Lift your buttocks into the air and pass the ball underneath with your right hand to the left side of your body.

Lower your buttocks to the floor and move the ball back to the starting position. Breathe as you lift and lower your buttocks. Complete your number of repetitions, then change direction.

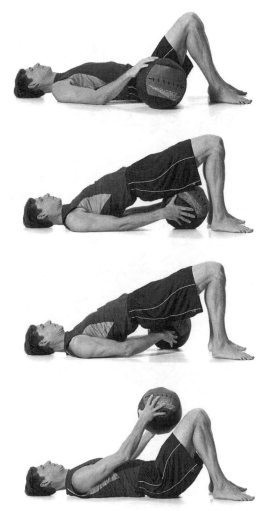

Three Way Hip

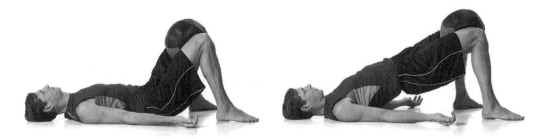

Lie on the floor on your back. Bend your knees and place your feet flat on the floor. Hold the ball between your thighs and knees, and raise your hips into the air. Try to create a straight line between your upper body and your thighs so that your body forms a "bridge." Pushing your hips up higher could strain your lower back, and not bringing them high enough will not provide the necessary flexibility needed for proper alignment.

Now, rhythmically squeeze and relax your grip on the ball with your thighs. Exhale with every squeeze of the ball.

Sit Up and Reach

Lie on the floor on your back, holding the ball on your chest and gripping it firmly with both hands. Bending your knees slightly, sit up slowly. Once you reach a seated position, straighten your knees. While you are sitting up, straighten your arms and extend the ball toward your feet, keeping the ball between chest and shoulder height. Continue to lean forward until you feel a stretch behind your thighs.

Now, slowly lower your weight back to the floor, rolling your back onto the floor one vertebra at a time until you are back on the floor. Be sure to keep your arms straight as you lower yourself. Set the ball back on your chest to complete the technique.

Exhale as you sit up and reach out, and again as you roll back to the floor.

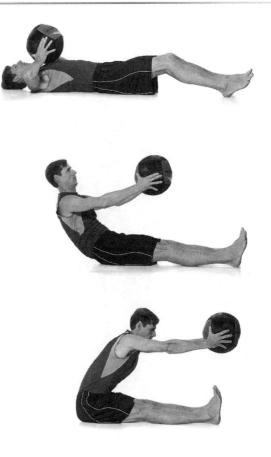

Twist and Sweep

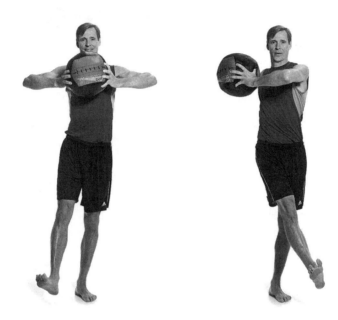

Start by standing on your left foot, with your right foot lifted a few inches in front of you. Hold the ball in front of your chest with your elbows pointing outward. Twist your upper chest (and the ball) to the right while sweeping your right foot to the left. Your pelvis should stay stationary and your abdominals and lower back should control the motion—but only your chest and leg should move.

During this motion, your leg remains straight and your foot stays pointed forward. Imagine putting a golf ball with your instep, then the outer edge of your foot, as your foot sweeps from side to side. Breathe out as you twist in either direction. Complete all repetitions on one side, then switch sides.

Straddle Squat and Reach

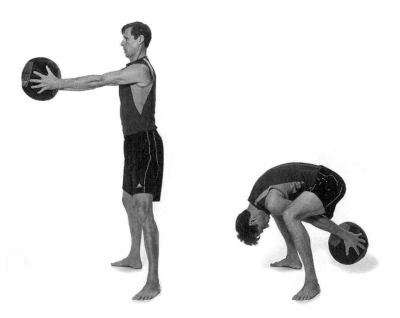

Begin with your feet parallel, but spaced very far apart. Your toes should be pointed outward. Press your big toes into the floor. Hold the ball at arm's length in front of your chest with both hands. Squat down, lean forward, and push the ball between your legs as far back as possible. This time, allow your entire back to become rounded as you push the ball, so that you feel a good stretch in your lower back.

Exhale as you reach down, again as you hold the final position, and again as you stand up. Return to the starting point to finish the repetition.

Squat and Hold

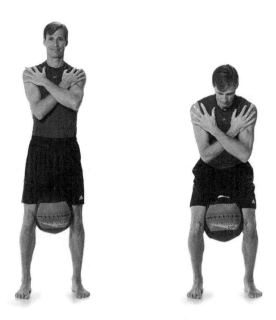

Stand in a parallel stance and place the ball between your knees and thighs, gripping it tightly between your legs. Cross your arms across your chest, lean forward slightly from your hips, and squat down halfway. Make sure to bend your hips and knees, not just your back. Keep your feet firmly planted on the floor, with more weight on the balls of your feet. Rhythmically squeeze and relax your grip on the ball with your legs. Breathe out with each squeeze.

Adapting *Four Way Burn* for Your Needs

Situp, Knee Lift, and Twist

Lie on your back on the floor with your feet straight in front of you, holding the ball on your chest and gripping it firmly with both hands. Sit up, rolling your weight down each vertebra of your spine as you lift yourself up. While you sit up, pull your right knee to your chest and turn your upper body to the right side. Do this move as if you were going to pass the ball to somebody behind you.

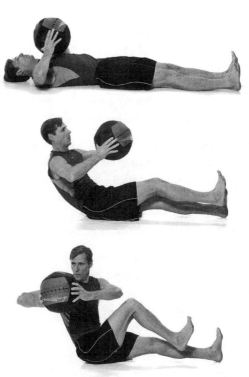

Turn until you feel the stretch, then return your upper body back to center and lower yourself, with control, back to the floor. Breathe out while you sit up and again when you lie down.

If lying on the floor with your feet straight causes lower back discomfort, bend your knees about 45 degrees to reduce the strain on your lower back.

Sit Up and Pass the Ball

Lie on your back on the floor with your legs straight out in front of you, firmly holding the ball with both hands against your chest. Sit up, rolling your weight down your spine as you lift yourself up. As you sit up, lift one leg off the floor, keeping it as straight as possible. Pass the ball under that leg from one hand to the other, then back.

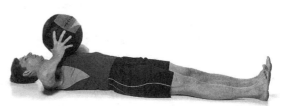

Lower your torso and leg back to the floor. On the next repetition, lift the same leg but change the direction in which you pass the ball from hand to hand. Exhale once sitting up, again as you pass the ball in each direction, and again as you lower yourself. Complete your repetitions, then switch to the other leg.

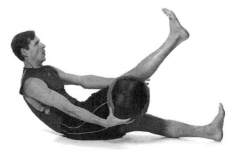

If lying on the floor causes discomfort in your back, bend your knees about 45 degrees to reduce strain on your lower back.

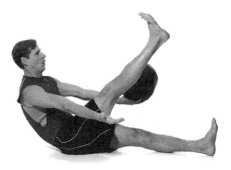

Adapting *Four Way Burn* for Your Needs

Good Morning with Side Twist

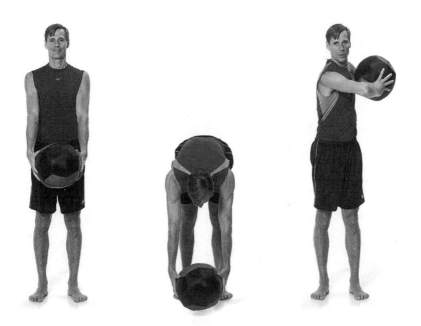

Begin with your feet parallel and closer than shoulder-width apart. At the starting position, hold the ball downward in front of your groin with your arms fully extended.

Lean straight down and touch the ball to the floor in front of your feet. Now, stand up while bringing the ball to your chest, and fully twist your torso to one side. While twisting, make sure that your elbows don't drop below chest level. Return your torso so that you're facing center to complete the repetition. Alternate between twisting left and right with each repetition.

Exhale as you bend down and as you twist.

Squat and Push

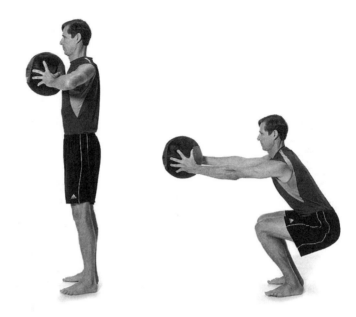

Begin in a parallel stance, holding the ball in front of your chest with your elbows pointed outward. Squat down as low as you can, or until your thighs are parallel to the floor, and fully extend the ball away from you until your arms are straightened in a soft lock. Look straight ahead at all times.

As you squat, keep your feet flat—don't rise up on your toes. As you stand up, simultaneously pull the ball back to your chest and squeeze your shoulder blades together.

Take in one deep breath going down, exhale, and take in another deep breath coming up.

Adapting *Four Way Burn* for Your Needs

Knee Tuck and Push

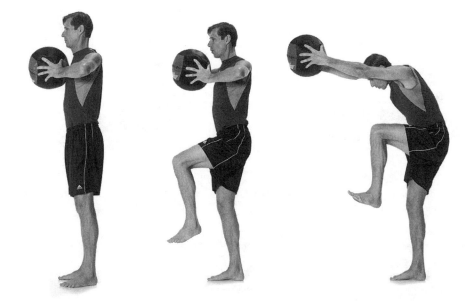

Begin in a parallel stance with your feet a few inches apart, holding the ball in front of your chest with your elbows pointed outward.

Lift one thigh upward until it's higher than parallel with the floor, keeping your foot flexed. At the same time, lean your upper body forward and extend your arms in a soft lock so the ball is held out from your body. It's okay to lower your head and hunch forward as you press the ball outward. Put more weight on the ball of the foot that you're standing on.

To complete the repetition, lower your foot and straighten that leg. Stand upright, and bring the ball back to your chest, keeping your elbows between chest and shoulder height and pulling your shoulder blades together. Exhale once as you push the ball away from you and again as you pull it back. Complete all repetitions on one side, then switch sides and repeat.

Single-Leg Raise and Crunch

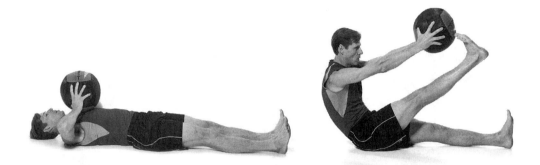

Lie on the floor on your back, with both legs extended and your ankles flexed. Grip the ball tightly between both hands, against your chest, with your elbows pointed out. Sit up, rolling your weight down your spine as you lift yourself up. At the same time, lift your right leg up—keeping it straight—and push the ball out toward the toes on your right foot, reaching as far as you can. You should feel the stretch in your hamstring. Complete the repetitions and change legs.

Breathe out as you crunch up and again as you lower yourself.

Seated Pass to Yourself

Sit on the floor with your knees bent and your heels touching the floor, and hold the ball with both hands on the right side of your hip. Lean back until you feel your abdominal muscles tightening. Keep both buttocks firmly on the floor. Roll the ball behind your body and to the left until you can't turn anymore. Leave the ball where it is, turn your upper body to your left, and grab the ball with both hands. Pass the ball back to your front, pick it up, and start it again on your right side. Finish the repetitions, then reverse the direction. Breathe out while turning in both directions.

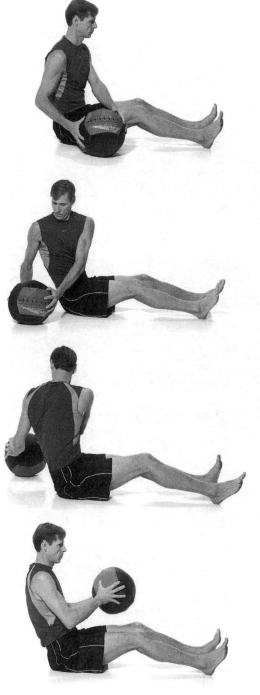

BACK PROGRAM CHART

CYCLE ONE

DAYS 1 AND 2

	Beginner	Intermediate	Advanced
Seated Side Twist	5 reps	8 reps	10 reps
Seated Good Morning	5 reps	8 reps	10 reps

Repeat the first two techniques for a second set, then move on to the next techniques.

	Beginner	Intermediate	Advanced
Wall Squat	20 sec	30 sec	40 sec
Reach, Tuck, and Touch	5 reps	8 reps	10 reps
Lying Side Twist	5 reps	8 reps	10 reps

Repeat the second group of techniques for a second set, then do the stretching/relaxation moves below (see pages 41 to 43).

Wedge
Lying Side Twist
Spread Eagle

DAYS 3 AND 4

	Beginner	Intermediate	Advanced
Seated Side Twist	7 reps	10 reps	12 reps
Seated Good Morning	7 reps	10 reps	12 reps

Repeat the first two techniques for a second set, then move on to the next techniques.

	Beginner	Intermediate	Advanced
Wall Squat	25 sec	35 sec	45 sec
Reach, Tuck, and Touch	7 reps	10 reps	12 reps
Lying Side Twist	7 reps	10 reps	12 reps

Repeat the second group of techniques for a second set, then do the stretching/relaxation moves below (see pages 41 to 43).

Wedge
Lying Side Twist
Spread Eagle

DAYS 5 AND 6

	Beginner	Intermediate	Advanced
Seated Side Twist	9 reps	12 reps	15 reps
Seated Good Morning	9 reps	12 reps	15 reps

Repeat the first two techniques for a second set, then move on to the next techniques.

	Beginner	Intermediate	Advanced
Wall Squat	30 sec	40 sec	50 sec
Reach, Tuck, and Touch	9 reps	12 reps	15 reps
Lying Side Twist	9 reps	12 reps	15 reps

Repeat the second group of techniques for a second set, then do the stretching/relaxation moves below (see pages 41 to 43).

Wedge
Lying Side Twist
Spread Eagle

CYCLE TWO

DAYS 1 AND 2

	Beginner	Intermediate	Advanced
Side Twist	5 reps	8 reps	10 reps
Squat and Reach	5 reps	8 reps	10 reps

Repeat the first two techniques for a second set, then move on to the next techniques.

	Beginner	Intermediate	Advanced
Bridging	5 reps	8 reps	10 reps
Three Way Hip	5 reps	8 reps	10 reps
Sit Up and Reach	5 reps	8 reps	10 reps

Repeat the second group of techniques for a second set, then do the stretching/relaxation moves below (see pages 41 to 43).

Wedge
Lying Side Twist
Spread Eagle

DAYS 3 AND 4

	Beginner	Intermediate	Advanced
Side Twist	7 reps	10 reps	12 reps
Squat and Reach	7 reps	10 reps	12 reps

Repeat the first two techniques for a second set, then move on to the next techniques.

	Beginner	Intermediate	Advanced
Bridging	7 reps	10 reps	12 reps
Three Way Hip	7 reps	10 reps	12 reps
Sit Up and Reach	7 reps	10 reps	12 reps

Repeat the second group of techniques for a second set, then do the stretching/relaxation moves below (see pages 41 to 43).

Wedge
Lying Side Twist
Spread Eagle

DAYS 5 AND 6

	Beginner	Intermediate	Advanced
Side Twist	9 reps	12 reps	15 reps
Squat and Reach	9 reps	12 reps	15 reps

Repeat the first two techniques for a second set, then move on to the next techniques.

	Beginner	Intermediate	Advanced
Bridging	9 reps	12 reps	15 reps
Three Way Hip	9 reps	12 reps	15 reps
Sit Up and Reach	9 reps	12 reps	15 reps

Repeat the second group of techniques for a second set, then do the stretching/relaxation moves below (see pages 41 to 43).

Wedge
Lying Side Twist
Spread Eagle

CYCLE ONE
DAY 7

	Beginner	Intermediate	Advanced
Seated Side Twist	12 reps	15 reps	20 reps
Seated Good Morning	12 reps	15 reps	20 reps
Repeat the first two techniques for a second set, then move on to the next techniques.			
Wall Squat	35 sec	45 sec	55 sec
Reach, Tuck, and Touch	12 reps	15 reps	20 reps
Lying Side Twist	12 reps	15 reps	20 reps
Repeat the second group of techniques for a second set, then do the stretching/relaxation moves below (see pages 41 to 43).			
Wedge			
Lying Side Twist			
Spread Eagle			

CYCLE THREE
DAYS 1 AND 2

	Beginner	Intermediate	Advanced
Twist and Sweep	7 reps	9 reps	12 reps
Straddle Squat and Reach	7 reps	9 reps	12 reps
Repeat the first two techniques for a second set, then move on to the next techniques.			
Squat and Hold	7 reps	9 reps	12 reps
Situp, Knee Lift, and Twist	7 reps	9 reps	12 reps
Sit Up and Pass the Ball	7 reps	9 reps	12 reps
Repeat the second group of techniques for a second set, then do the stretching/relaxation moves below (see pages 41 to 43).			
Wedge			
Lying Side Twist			
Spread Eagle			

DAYS 3 AND 4

	Beginner	Intermediate	Advanced
Twist and Sweep	9 reps	12 reps	15 reps
Straddle Squat and Reach	9 reps	12 reps	15 reps
Repeat the first two techniques for a second set, then move on to the next techniques.			
Squat and Hold	9 reps	12 reps	15 reps
Situp, Knee Lift, and Twist	9 reps	12 reps	15 reps
Sit Up and Pass the Ball	9 reps	12 reps	15 reps
Repeat the second group of techniques for a second set, then do the stretching/relaxation moves below (see pages 41 to 43).			
Wedge			
Lying Side Twist			
Spread Eagle			

CYCLE TWO
DAY 7

	Beginner	Intermediate	Advanced
Side Twist	12 reps	15 reps	20 reps
Squat and Reach	12 reps	15 reps	20 reps
Repeat the first two techniques for a second set, then move on to the next techniques.			
Bridging	12 reps	15 reps	20 reps
Three Way Hip	12 reps	15 reps	20 reps
Sit Up and Reach	12 reps	15 reps	20 reps
Repeat the second group of techniques for a second set, then do the stretching/relaxation moves below (see pages 41 to 43).			
Wedge			
Lying Side Twist			
Spread Eagle			

CYCLE FOUR
DAYS 1 AND 2

	Beginner	Intermediate	Advanced
Good Morning with Side Twist	7 reps	9 reps	12 reps
Squat and Push	7 reps	9 reps	12 reps
Repeat the first two techniques for a second set, then move on to the next techniques.			
Knee Tuck and Push	7 reps	9 reps	12 reps
Single-Leg Raise and Crunch	7 reps	9 reps	12 reps
Seated Pass to Yourself	7 reps	9 reps	12 reps
Repeat the second group of techniques for a second set, then do the stretching/relaxation moves below (see pages 41 to 43).			
Wedge			
Lying Side Twist			
Spread Eagle			

DAYS 3 AND 4

	Beginner	Intermediate	Advanced
Good Morning with Side Twist	9 reps	12 reps	15 reps
Squat and Push	9 reps	12 reps	15 reps
Repeat the first two techniques for a second set, then move on to the next techniques.			
Knee Tuck and Push	9 reps	12 reps	15 reps
Single-Leg Raise and Crunch	9 reps	12 reps	15 reps
Seated Pass to Yourself	9 reps	12 reps	15 reps
Repeat the second group of techniques for a second set, then do the stretching/relaxation moves below (see pages 41 to 43).			
Wedge			
Lying Side Twist			
Spread Eagle			

(continued)

BACK PROGRAM CHART (*cont.*)

CYCLE THREE

DAYS 5 AND 6

	Beginner	Intermediate	Advanced
Twist and Sweep	12 reps	15 reps	20 reps
Straddle Squat and Reach	12 reps	15 reps	20 reps
Repeat the first two techniques for a second set, then move on to the next techniques.			
Squat and Hold	12 reps	15 reps	20 reps
Situp, Knee Lift, and Twist	12 reps	15 reps	20 reps
Sit Up and Pass the Ball	12 reps	15 reps	20 reps
Repeat the second group of techniques for a second set, then do the stretching/relaxation moves below (see pages 41 to 43).			
Wedge			
Lying Side Twist			
Spread Eagle			

DAY 7

	Beginner	Intermediate	Advanced
Twist and Sweep	15 reps	20 reps	25 reps
Straddle Squat and Reach	15 reps	20 reps	25 reps
Repeat the first two techniques for a second set, then move on to the next techniques.			
Squat and Hold	15 reps	20 reps	25 reps
Situp, Knee Lift, and Twist	15 reps	20 reps	25 reps
Sit Up and Pass the Ball	15 reps	20 reps	25 reps
Repeat the second group of techniques for a second set, then do the stretching/relaxation moves below (see pages 41 to 43).			
Wedge			
Lying Side Twist			
Spread Eagle			

CYCLE FOUR

DAYS 5 AND 6

	Beginner	Intermediate	Advanced
Good Morning with Side Twist	12 reps	15 reps	20 reps
Squat and Push	12 reps	15 reps	20 reps
Repeat the first two techniques for a second set, then move on to the next techniques.			
Knee Tuck and Push	12 reps	15 reps	20 reps
Single-Leg Raise and Crunch	12 reps	15 reps	20 reps
Seated Pass to Yourself	12 reps	15 reps	20 reps
Repeat the second group of techniques for a second set, then do the stretching/relaxation moves below (see pages 41 to 43).			
Wedge			
Lying Side Twist			
Spread Eagle			

DAY 7

	Beginner	Intermediate	Advanced
Good Morning with Side Twist	15 reps	20 reps	25 reps
Squat and Push	15 reps	20 reps	25 reps
Repeat the first two techniques for a second set, then move on to the next techniques.			
Knee Tuck and Push	15 reps	20 reps	25 reps
Single-Leg Raise and Crunch	15 reps	20 reps	25 reps
Seated Pass to Yourself	15 reps	20 reps	25 reps
Repeat the second group of techniques for a second set, then do the stretching/relaxation moves below (see pages 41 to 43).			
Wedge			
Lying Side Twist			
Spread Eagle			

USING
FOUR WAY BURN
FOR PEAK
SPORTS
PERFORMANCE

10

GET READY FOR WALKING AND RUNNING WITH *FOUR WAY BURN*

Walking, jogging, and running are all very effective in helping you control your weight or shed extra pounds. Since these activities require you to carry your own body weight, they burn more calories than seated activities such as biking or rowing.

And, since they're weight-bearing exercises, these activities also help to keep your bones strong. However, gravity can be a foe as well as a friend. Working against it during physical activity keeps your body strong and fit—but too *much* weight-bearing activity, particularly if your body is out of alignment, can cause injury. It is important when you walk or run to:

- ► Make sure that you build strength and flexibility around your ankles, knees, lower back, and shoulder girdle so that they can handle the impact with the least amount of wear and tear.
- ► Use good posture and proper mechanics so that the muscle groups used in walking and running work together properly.
- ► Slowly and gradually increase your mileage. For example, you shouldn't add more than 5 minutes to your walking or running time or 5 percent more distance during a session. Also, when you increase your time or distance, do at least three sessions before increasing again.

In order to prevent walking or running injuries—and to better develop the muscle groups that these activities require—I urge you to add the modified *Four Way Burn* program offered in this chapter to your walking or running program. Before we get to the program, though, let's look at how your body should move when you walk or run.

THE BASIC MECHANICS OF WALKING AND JOGGING

What body parts do you use when you walk or jog? You'd probably think of your legs first. You do use your legs, of course, but you also utilize your arms, upper body, and core muscles to control and counterbalance your legs in motion. Without all these muscle groups working properly, you won't do well in these activities.

Your upper body. Moving with your head tilted down or with your shoulders rounded produces tremendous strain on your upper back. This may result in problems with your spine, your hips, and even your knees.

Your hips. The hip flexors, located at the top of the thigh, initiate your leg movement, and they actually lift the leg off the ground. Strong hip flexors are important for long and powerful strides. People with weak hip flexors often shuffle their legs, and they also have a hard time climbing stairs and usually have bad balance. Improving the strength in your hip flexors will also aid in trail walking and quickly stepping over obstacles.

Your hips also provide the base upon which your spine rests. The muscles that you think of as the buttocks (the gluteus maximus muscles) don't have the strength to support the spine. Two smaller buttock muscles behind and below the hip—the gluteus minimus and gluteus medius—are responsible for keeping your hips stable and for supporting the weight of your spine and upper body. If you sway from side to side when you walk, it's a good indicator that these muscles need to be strengthened and integrated as part of an overall conditioning program.

Your hamstrings. These muscles behind your thighs are particularly vulnerable to strain. Ideally, your hamstrings should have the proper strength and flexibility to balance out the muscles on the front of your thighs. However, many of us have tight and shortened hamstrings because of our sedentary jobs or lifestyles. Lengthening and strengthening your hamstrings will improve your stride length and allow for a faster, more powerful pace.

Your quadriceps. One muscle that's important for stabilizing and supporting the knee, but that is often overlooked, is the vastus medialis oblique (VMO). It's one of the quadriceps muscles on the front of your thigh. Smooth tracking or gliding of the knee while it's in motion is important to prevent premature wearing of the soft tissue behind the kneecap, as well as other injuries. However, this muscle fires best when you fully extend your leg, and most people (especially men) have a hard time straightening their legs completely because of tight hamstrings.

Again, balancing these opposing muscles with the right amount of strength and flexibility will help protect your knees from wear and tear.

Your knees. These joints are constantly challenged from the force below as your feet hit the ground, as you move over uneven surfaces, as you change directions, and from the weight of your body above. Proper positioning and correct alignment of your head, shoulder girdle, spine, pelvis, and feet will help you distribute these natural forces proportionately around your knees. And strengthening the muscles you don't see—the ones on the back side of your body—will also help to ensure better balance.

Your feet. Your feet are the only body parts that touch the ground, and it's important that they land properly. Proper foot alignment and placement will help to better distribute the impact on your lower legs. Sprained or strained ankles, pain in the sole of the foot, toe problems, shinsplints, strained Achilles tendons, and knee injuries can indicate improper alignment or weakness of the feet.

In addition to transferring impact well, it's important to have strong, flexible feet since your feet and toes contain an elaborate sensory system that sends information to your central nervous system. Your nervous system uses this information to quickly adjust your body so that it stays balanced. Imbalance in your feet can cause imbalance in the rest of your body.

THE *FOUR WAY BURN* WALKING AND JOGGING PROGRAM

A month before you start walking or jogging frequently, go through the following special 4-week *Four Way Burn* program to get conditioned for these activities. Then, during times of the year when you're walking or jogging a lot, keep doing these sessions on your "off" days.

During the rest of the year, switch back to the regular program that forms the bulk of this book.

You'll do three sessions per week. Each session contains five techniques. Do the first two, then repeat them for a second set. Move on to the next three techniques, then repeat them for a second set. The repetitions you should do are listed in the chart on page 173.

Each session should take 20 to 30 minutes, depending on whether you do it at the beginner, intermediate, or advanced level. To help determine which level to do, consult the chart on pages 28 and 29.

The Elements of Good Walking and Running Form

Running differs from walking in that it requires you to have only one foot in contact with the ground at any time.

However, in both running and walking, you must maintain a balanced and upright posture. Thus, the form for walking and running (or jogging, which is a slow form of running) follows the same basic principles.

To get yourself into proper walking, running, or jogging form, keep these 12 principles in mind.

- ▶ Keep your head up and your pelvis in the "suck and tuck" position, with your trunk and head directly above your hips.

- ▶ Let your arms hang loosely at the sides of your body.

- ▶ Make fists, with your thumbs up or resting across your index and middle fingers. Walking or running with your hands in fists makes you pay better attention to the position of your upper body, head, and shoulders. When people run with their hands open, they often have bad form, with their shoulders and head drooping.

- ▶ Lean forward slightly, bending your ankles until your body weight is more toward the balls of your feet.

- ▶ Bend your elbows to create a 90-degree angle between your lower and upper arms.

- ▶ Lift your heel and push off with the ball of your foot.

- ▶ Bend your leg at the knee and drive it forward.

- ▶ Bring your foot forward under your knee.

- ▶ Strike the ground with your heel, with your foot landing on the ground under your body, not ahead of it.

- ▶ Swing your arms forward and back, without using your shoulder muscles. Keep your shoulders relaxed and parallel to the ground.

- ▶ Focus on keeping a "tall" posture.

- ▶ Keep your upper body facing forward—not twisted to the side.

The Coil

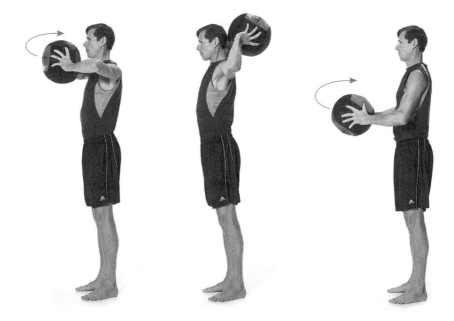

To begin, start in the Saturn position (see page 32). Move the ball around your head, then smoothly lower it and pass it around your midsection. As the ball comes back around to your abdomen, squat down and pass it behind your legs and back in front of you. Now keep moving the ball up and around your body in a

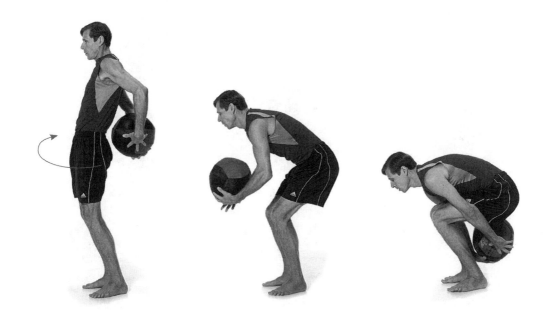

Hula Hoop (see page 36) and a Saturn until it ends in front of your face. Going all the way down and all the way up is one repetition. Exhale as the ball passes in front of you each time. Complete all repetitions in one direction, then switch directions and repeat.

Golfer Swing

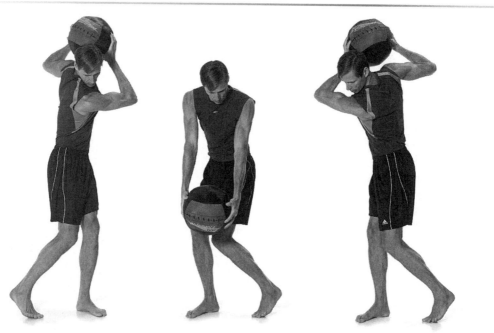

Begin with your feet positioned parallel and less than shoulder-width apart. Extend your arms and hold the ball in front of your groin. Bring the ball with both hands up to one shoulder, as if you're setting up to swing a golf club. Just before you make this motion, start pivoting your feet so that they point toward the direction in which the ball is traveling. Your entire body will be pivoting as you bring the ball above your shoulder. At the highest point, bend both elbows.

When you reach your highest point and have finished the upward motion, pivot your feet the other way and move the ball back down, across your groin and up to your other shoulder. Your arms and the ball will look like a pendulum swinging down and up from shoulder to shoulder as your feet pivot back and forth. Exhale forcefully with each swing. Complete all repetitions on one side, then switch sides and repeat.

Around the World

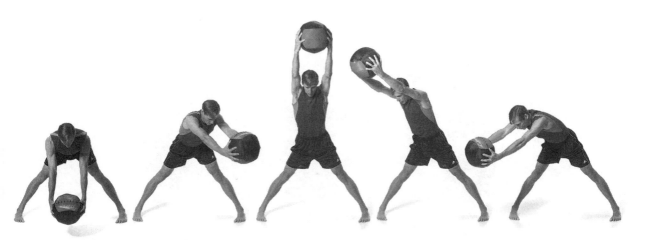

Begin with your feet in a parallel stance, spaced farther than shoulder-width apart. Keep your legs straight, with your toes pointed inward and pressed into the floor.

Lean forward deeply and hold the ball toward the floor in both hands with your arms fully extended. Reaching out as far as you can, move the ball out to your left and up until it's overhead, and on to your right and back down to the starting point. As you reach the high point of this circle, stretch yourself up as tall as you can. Keep your arms and legs straight as you make the circle. Finish all repetitions in one direction, then switch directions.

Exhale as your hands travel past each quarter of the circle.

Crossover Stand and Reach

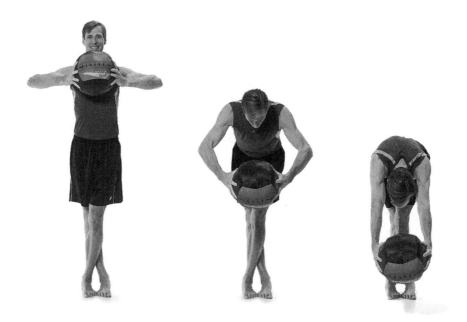

Stand with your feet crossed over each other, so that each is flat on the floor and next to the other, but on opposite sides. Hold the ball with both hands at chest level. Anchor your feet by pressing your big toes into the floor.

Bend over at the hips and reach out as far as you can with the ball toward the floor and straight away from your feet, keeping your legs straight at all times.

Breathe out fully on the way down and again when you return to the starting position. Repeat until you've completed the required repetitions, then switch sides and repeat.

Squat and One-Arm Reach

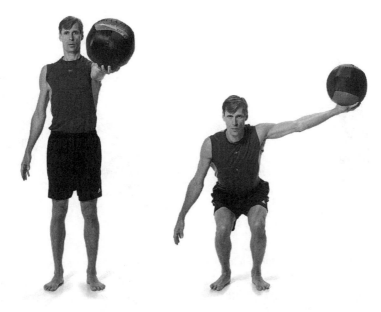

Begin with your feet parallel but spaced shoulder-width apart. Your toes should be pointed outward. Press your big toes into the floor to anchor your feet. Hold the ball in your left hand at arm's length in front of your chest.

Squat down and extend the ball forward and out toward the left at an angle away from your body. The ball should never drop below shoulder level. Exhale as you reach out, then briefly hold the final position and return to the starting point to finish the repetition. Do all the repetitions with your left arm, then repeat with your right.

Back Lunge, Push, Pull, and Side Twist

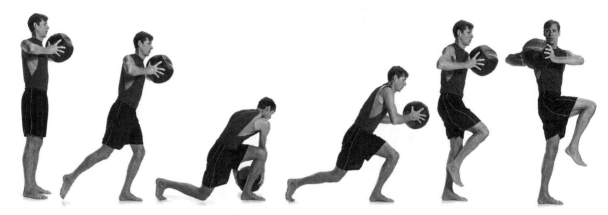

Stand with your feet in a parallel stance a few inches apart, holding the ball firmly in your hands at chest level, with your elbows out to the sides. Lunge back with your right leg. Lower your right knee close to the floor and bend your left knee. Keep your left knee squarely above your left ankle. Now, lean over your left thigh and touch the floor with the ball, keeping a firm grip on it with both hands.

With your body weight shifting to your left foot, stand up and draw your right knee upward so that you're balancing on your left leg. Push the ball out until your arms are fully extended in a soft lock, then pull it back to your chest. Keep a firm grip throughout the motion. While still balancing on the left leg with your right knee lifted and the ball at your chest, twist your upper body to the right side. Your hips and legs should remain facing forward, while your upper body twists sideways. Turn back to the starting position to finish the repetition. Complete your repetitions, then switch to the other leg. Breathe out six times: when lunging back, coming up, pushing and pulling, and twisting to the right and again when you come back to center.

Soldier Walk

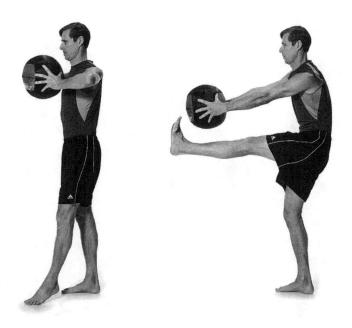

Begin with most of your weight on one foot and the other lightly touching the floor in front of you. Grip the ball in front of your chest with your elbows pointed outward. Lift your front leg up while keeping it fully extended. At the same time, push the ball straight out and touch it to your lower shin when your leg reaches its maximum height. Exhale as you touch the ball to your shin.

Keeping your leg fully straightened, lower your foot back to the floor while you pull the ball back to your chest. Finish your repetitions with one foot, then switch feet.

Pecking Bird

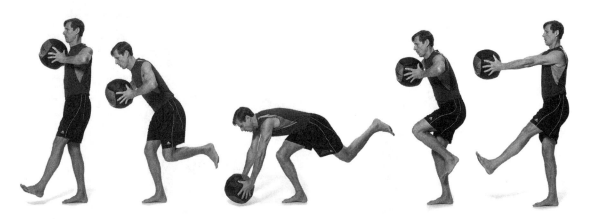

Stand on one foot, with your other leg extended in front of you and that foot raised a few inches off the floor. Hold the ball at chest level with your elbows out. Slowly lean forward, extend your arms, and touch the ball to the floor (or reach as far as you can). As you're leaning over, do a mini-squat on your standing leg, and bring your front leg back behind you, bending it at the knee. Straighten back up and push the ball out at chest level, simultaneously bringing your rear leg back out to the front. Complete all your repetitions on that leg, then switch legs and repeat.

Exhale four times—when you lean and squat down, stand back up, push the ball out, and pull it back to your chest.

Good Morning with Side Twist

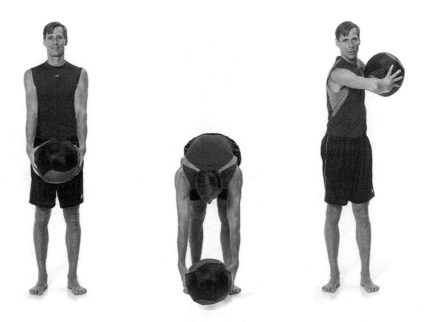

Begin with your feet parallel and closer than shoulder-width apart. At the starting position, hold the ball downward in front of your groin with your arms fully extended.

Lean straight down and touch the ball to the floor in front of your feet. Now, stand up while bringing the ball to your chest, and fully twist your torso to one side. While twisting, make sure your elbows don't drop below chest level. Return your torso so that you're facing center to complete the repetition. Alternate between twisting left and right with each repetition.

Exhale as you bend down and as you twist.

Triceps and Leg Extensions

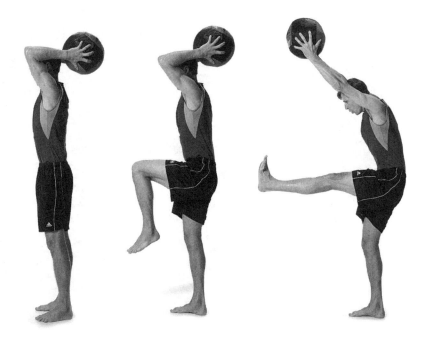

Begin in a parallel stance with your feet just a few inches apart. "Suck and tuck" your pelvis. Hold the ball with both hands behind the back of your neck, keeping your elbows close to your head. Lift one leg until your thigh is parallel with the floor, and extend your foot until your leg is straight. You should feel the stretch behind your thigh. At the same time, bring the ball over your head and forward until your arms are fully extended at an upward angle toward the ceiling. Return to the starting position to complete the repetition. Alternate feet with each repetition.

Exhale when you reach out with the ball and again when you pull it back.

Carioca Loop

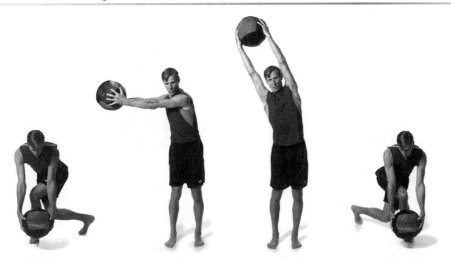

Begin by squatting down with most of your weight on your left leg, and your right foot touching the floor behind you and out to your left. Both knees should be bent and your right foot should rest on the ball of that foot. Lean forward, fully extend your arms, and let the ball hang to your left knee.

Keeping your arms fully extended, bring the ball in a wide circle toward the right, then overhead, while at the same time stepping up with your back foot into a parallel stance. You should reach this stance just as the ball reaches the point straight overhead. Continue moving the ball in a circle toward the left and down as you step behind with your left foot. You will end up with most of your weight on your right leg, with your left leg behind you and out to your right, and your arms fully extended and holding the ball just below your right knee. This is the mirror opposite of how you started. Exhale while you're lifting and lowering the ball. Complete all repetitions in this direction, then switch directions and repeat.

Knee Lift and Side Twist

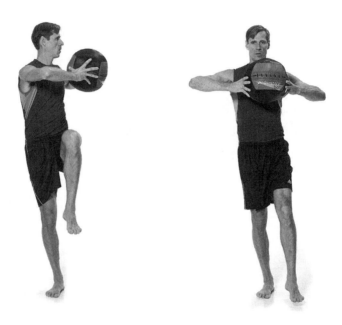

Start with your feet parallel and closer than shoulder-width apart. Hold the ball in front of your chest with your elbows pointing out to the side. Twist your torso all the way to the left while you raise your left thigh until it's parallel with the floor.

As you set your foot back down, twist your torso all the way to the right. Return your torso to center to complete the repetition. Breathe out as you twist in each direction.

Split Squat and Pass

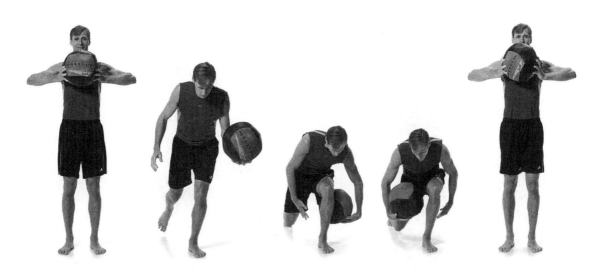

Stand up straight in a parallel stance, holding the ball firmly in your hands at chest level.

Lunge back with your right leg. Lower your right knee close to the floor and bend your left knee. Keep your left knee squarely above the left ankle. Lean over your left thigh and pass the ball beneath the thigh from your left hand to the right and then back to the left hand. Stand back up. Repeat, but this time pass the ball from your right hand to your left hand.

Alternate until you finish your repetitions, then repeat with the opposite leg. Breathe out four times: as you lunge back, pass in each direction, and stand up.

Hop and Twist

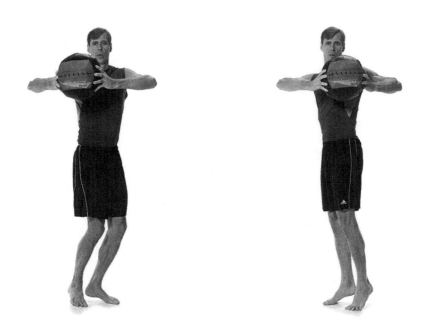

Hold the ball firmly in both hands and higher than chest level. Stand with most of your weight on the balls of your feet. "Suck and tuck" your pelvis by pulling in your belly button and tightening your buttocks.

Now, hop in one place and simultaneously twist your hips from one direction to the other. Keep a tight grip on the ball. Exhale with each hop.

Rocking Chair

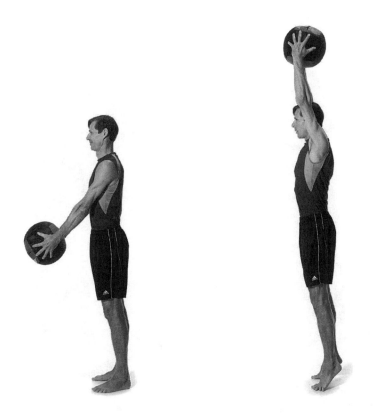

Begin with your feet in a parallel stance, spaced less than shoulder-width apart. Stand up straight and hold the ball so that it's hanging down in front of your groin with your arms fully extended.

Rise up on your toes as you bring the ball straight overhead. Your arms should remain fully extended—never bending—at all times. If you can't bring the ball straight overhead, go as high as your flexibility allows. Now, lower the ball back to the starting position as you rock back onto your heels.

Breathe out as you rock on your feet in each direction.

Twist and Sweep

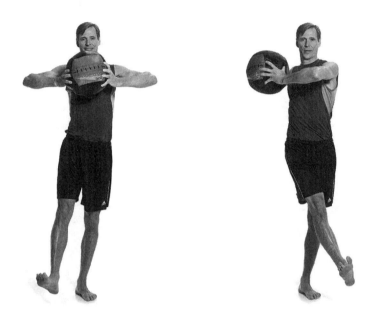

Start by standing on your left foot, with your right foot lifted a few inches in front of you. Hold the ball in front of your chest with your elbows pointing outward. Twist your upper chest (and the ball) to the right while sweeping your right foot to the left. Your pelvis should stay stationary and your abdominals and lower back should control the motion—but only your chest and leg should move.

During this motion, your leg should remain straight and your foot should stay pointed forward. Imagine putting a golf ball with your instep, then the outer edge of your foot, as your foot sweeps from side to side. Breathe out as you twist in either direction. Complete all repetitions on one side, then switch sides.

Side Bend

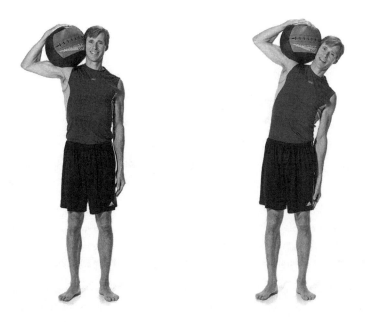

Stand tall in a parallel stance. Hold the ball between your right ear and your right shoulder by holding it tightly with your right arm. Your right elbow should point out to the side.

"Suck and tuck" your pelvis. Now, bend your upper body to the left side, making sure not to move your lower body or twist your upper body. Slide your left fingertips down your left thigh while you are bending in that direction. Keep your head straight. After completing your repetitions to the left, switch to the right side. Breathe out as you bend in each direction.

Spider Walk

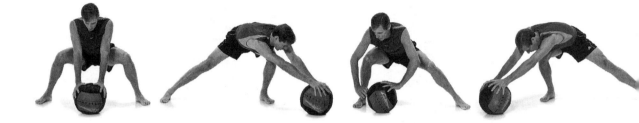

Begin with your feet in a parallel stance but spaced more than shoulder-width apart. Set the ball on the floor so that you're straddling it, and place both hands on the ball. Bend your knees and lower your buttocks until your thighs are parallel to the floor, and dig into the floor with your big toes.

With both hands, roll the ball out to the left away from you as far as you can go. Roll it back to the center, then out to the right to complete one repetition. Take two breaths while rolling the ball in each direction.

Front-Arm Raise with Leg Abduction

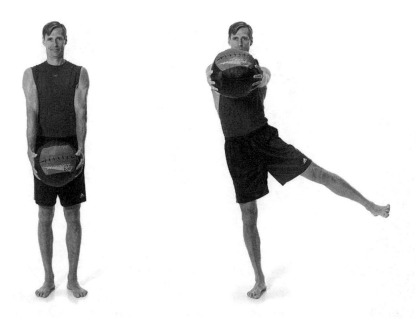

Stand in a parallel stance with your shoulder-width apart. Hold the ball in both hands with a strong grip and your arms fully extended so that the ball is in front of your groin. Lift one leg out to the side while lifting the ball upward until your arms are parallel to the floor, keeping your arms and legs fully extended. To complete the repetition, lower your arms to the starting position and lower your foot until your heels touch. Complete all repetitions, then switch sides and repeat.

Exhale when lifting the ball and again when lowering it.

Thigh Kick and Catch with 90-Degree-Turn Jumps

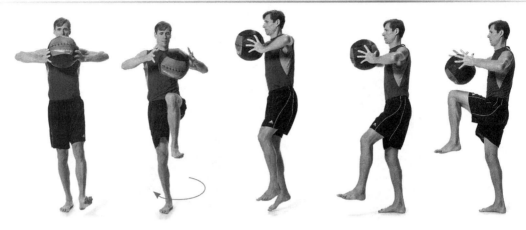

Hold the ball firmly in both hands and higher than chest level. Stand on one leg, with most of your weight on the ball of your foot, and raise your other leg until your thigh is parallel to the floor.

Drop the ball onto your thigh, kick it with your thigh, then catch it as it bounces up. Hop and swivel a quarter-turn to the right.

Breathe out with each kick and each hop. Keep repeating until you turn all the way around. After completion, change legs. When you've done both legs, switch legs again and repeat, this time reversing the direction of your rotation. That equals one repetition.

WALKING/RUNNING CONDITIONING CHART

WEEK 1

	Beginner	Intermediate	Advanced
The Coil	10 reps each direction	15 reps each direction	20 reps each direction
Golfer Swing	10 reps each direction	15 reps each direction	20 reps each direction

Repeat the first two techniques for a second set, then move on to the next techniques.

	Beginner	Intermediate	Advanced
Around the World	5 reps each direction	8 reps each direction	10 reps each direction
Crossover Stand and Reach	10 reps each direction	15 reps each direction	20 reps each direction
Squat and One-Arm Reach	5 reps each direction	8 reps each direction	10 reps each direction

Repeat the second group of techniques for a second set, then do the stretching/relaxation moves below (see pages 41 to 43).

Wedge
Lying Side Twist
Spread Eagle

WEEK 2

	Beginner	Intermediate	Advanced
Back Lunge, Push, Pull, and Side Twist	6 reps each leg	8 reps each leg	12 reps each leg
Soldier Walk	10 reps each leg	15 reps each leg	20 reps each leg

Repeat the first two techniques for a second set, then move on to the next techniques.

	Beginner	Intermediate	Advanced
Pecking Bird	5 reps each leg	8 reps each leg	10 reps each leg
Good Morning with Side Twist	10 reps each side	15 reps each side	20 reps each side
Triceps and Leg Extensions	10 reps each leg	15 reps each leg	20 reps each leg

Repeat the second group of techniques for a second set, then do the stretching/relaxation moves below (see pages 41 to 43).

Wedge
Lying Side Twist
Spread Eagle

WEEK 3

	Beginner	Intermediate	Advanced
Carioca Loop	5 reps each direction	8 reps each direction	10 reps each direction
Knee Lift and Side Twist	10 reps each side	15 reps each side	20 reps each side

Repeat the first two techniques for a second set, then move on to the next techniques.

	Beginner	Intermediate	Advanced
Split Squat and Pass	6 reps each direction	10 reps each direction	14 reps each direction
Hop and Twist	10 reps each direction	15 reps each direction	20 reps each direction
Rocking Chair	10 reps	15 reps	20 reps

Repeat the second group of techniques for a second set, then do the stretching/relaxation moves below (see pages 41 to 43).

Wedge
Lying Side Twist
Spread Eagle

WEEK 4

	Beginner	Intermediate	Advanced
Twist and Sweep	10 reps each direction	15 reps each direction	20 reps each direction
Side Bend	10 reps each direction	15 reps each direction	20 reps each direction

Repeat the first two techniques for a second set, then move on to the next techniques.

	Beginner	Intermediate	Advanced
Spider Walk	5 reps each direction	10 reps each direction	15 reps each direction
Front-Arm Raise with Leg Abduction	5 reps each direction	10 reps each direction	15 reps each direction
Thigh Kick and Catch with 90-Degree-Turn Jumps	4 reps each leg and each direction	6 reps each leg and each direction	8 reps each leg and each direction

Repeat the second group of techniques for a second set, then do the stretching/relaxation moves below (see pages 41 to 43).

Wedge
Lying Side Twist
Spread Eagle

11

GOOD FORM KEEPS A CYCLIST'S BODY ROLLING ALONG

Three or four times a week, you can find me riding my favorite 40-mile loops on my bicycle in the rolling hills around my home. Bicycling is an excellent activity for conditioning your cardiovascular system, and it makes a great component for a cross-training program when combined with other activities such as running, swimming, and the *Four Way Burn* program.

In addition, cycling strengthens your thighs, and because you're sitting upright and leaned forward for long periods, it also helps stretch your lower back and improves its muscular endurance.

However, bicycling can cause soreness and injuries if you're not properly prepared for it. Because you are leaning forward for an extended period of time, you may have some back pain. And since you make a lot of repetitive motions with many muscle groups and joints—in your calves, knees, and hips, of course, but also in your hands, wrists, neck, and shoulders—these may become "weak links" prone to injury.

To help reduce your risk of injuries, the program offered in this chapter will address any weaknesses you may have so that you can stay strong and fit for bicycling. Here's how *Four Way Burn* techniques can keep your entire body—and your mind—performing well while you're on your bike.

Your upper body. The importance of the upper body is often underestimated in biking. Your upper body must be resilient and strong to hold the handlebar and the front wheel steady. Also, when you need to rise out of your saddle to climb uphill, much of your weight shifts to your upper body, so you need to be able to support that weight.

You also need a strong neck and rear shoulder girdle to hold up your head, which is in a compromised position—sometimes for hours—while you lean forward and look ahead. And your forearms, hands, wrists, and fingers must be up to the task of constantly steering, maneuvering the gear levers, and braking.

Your trunk. The abdominal and back muscles are a weak link in most cyclists. That's not good. The force that you direct down into the pedals also travels upward into your torso. If your trunk is weak, the force that your powerful legs generate doesn't go down into the pedals, but is dissipated up into your torso instead. Riding with underdeveloped abdominals is like riding a bike with a cracked frame—all the energy gets wasted instead of moving you down the road.

Also, since every pedal stroke generates a pull in your back, if your lower back is not proportionately conditioned, your legs will overburden it and cause fatigue and spasms. In addition to strength, you also need suppleness in your lower back to lean over and hold an aerodynamic position for an extended period of time. You'll find that the techniques in this chapter provide this benefit, too.

Your buttocks and hips. These keep you firm and stable in the saddle. If you start rocking from one hip to the other, it could be an indicator that your buttocks and hips are too weak to give you the proper support. It could also mean that your saddle is not at the proper height, the frame of the bike is the wrong size for you, or you are not positioned over the bike properly.

Your thighs. The muscles of your thighs are constantly in use while cycling. Your quadriceps and hip flexors work to keep the pedals going in a circular motion. The quads push the pedals down and the hip flexors contract to pull your legs up.

In general, your quadriceps, which are found on the front of your thigh, become really strong from bicycling. However, one muscle in the quadriceps, called the vastus medialis oblique (VMO) muscle doesn't get much of a workout. It only flexes when your leg is extended nearly straight, but when you bicycle while sitting in the saddle, your legs are never straight. Having strong VMO muscles is invaluable for when you get out of the saddle and stand up on the pedals for more power. Strong VMOs also help prevent knee pain because they stabilize your knees and keep them from wobbling. That's why several techniques in this chapter require you to fully extend your legs. Strengthening the VMO muscles also strengthens the anterior cruciate ligament, which you need for standing up from the saddle.

Many cyclists are also not strong enough in the hip flexor muscles, so they predominantly use their thighs instead. This can lead to imbalances and eventually to injuries. Balancing these muscles with the correct strength ratio is essential for a fluid pedal stroke.

The hamstrings in the backs of your thighs are also important for powerful thigh movements. For a short time during each pedal stroke, your hamstrings help to power the stroke, which lets your quadriceps rest for a moment.

Finally, your thigh and groin muscles must work closely with your abdominal muscles during the pedal stroke. By making sure that they work well together, you help to ensure that the force of your legs is directed down into the pedals so that you move effectively.

Your calves and knees. These help cyclists stand up strong when climbing a hill or accelerating from a standing position. When your thighs are exhausted and you need just another short burst of energy to keep up with a group of riders or pull ahead of them, getting out of the saddle and standing up on the pedals is necessary to recruit that last bit of energy.

Your ankles and feet. Strong ankles and feet keep your shoes solid in the cleats. Weak ankles and feet make it harder to clip your shoes in or release them.

Your mind and senses. In addition to all the physical components needed for cycling, you also need excellent balance, vision, depth perception, and reaction time. This program will help you maintain the neuromuscular conditioning that you need to stay upright on your bicycle in a challenging environment with wet roads, changing road surfaces, low light, traffic signals, and intolerant drivers.

YOUR *FOUR WAY BURN* BICYCLING PROGRAM

During the off season or any other extended break from bicycling, the following program will not only help you maintain a good foundation for those early spring rides but will also help you avoid burnout when it's time to resume your tough training sessions later in the season.

Do the following 4-week program before you start riding regularly, such as in the very early spring before warm weather arrives. During each session, do the first two techniques, then repeat them for a second set, then do the next three and repeat those for a second set.

Later, during times when you're bicycling a lot, continue to do five techniques of your choice to maintain the benefits you have achieved. Do them for three sessions each week on days you're not riding, then the next week pick a different five techniques that you like.

Push and Pull

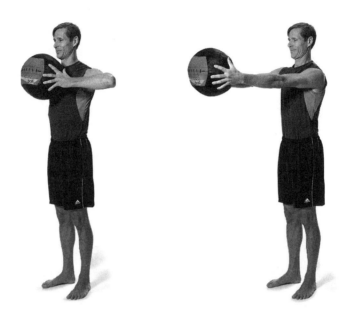

Begin in a parallel stance, with your feet side by side and spaced shoulder-width apart.

At the beginning of the motion, start by holding the ball at your chest with your elbows pointed out to the sides. Push the ball out until your arms are fully extended in a soft lock. On the first third of the repetitions, push the ball straight out. On the next third of the repetitions, push it out diagonally to your left. On the final third of the repetitions, push it out diagonally to your right. While pushing out at an angle, twist your upper body toward that particular side. Draw the ball back to your chest, and repeat.

Breathe out as you push the ball away from you, inhale, and breathe out again as you pull the ball toward you.

Saturn

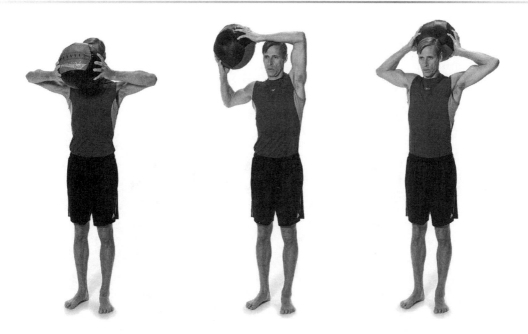

Stand in a parallel stance with your feet less than shoulder-width apart. Grip the ball in both hands in front of your face, with your elbows pointed outward. Now rotate the ball around your head in a circle. As it travels around your head, keep your elbows pointed outward. Breathe out for half of the circle around your head, and breathe in for the other half.

Do the recommended number of repetitions, then switch directions and repeat for the same number. All the repetitions in both directions equal one set.

Squat and Push

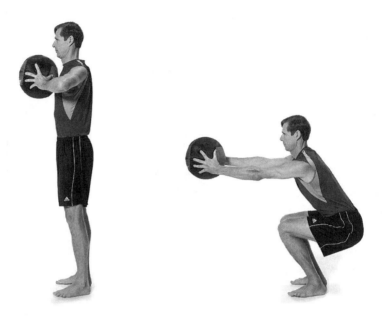

Begin in a parallel stance. Start by holding the ball in front of your chest with your elbows pointed outward. Now squat down. As you squat, fully extend the ball away from you until your arms are straightened in a soft lock. Look straight ahead at all times.

As you squat, keep your feet flat—don't rise up on your toes. As you stand up, simultaneously pull the ball back to your chest and squeeze your shoulder blades together. Take in one deep breath going down, exhale, and take in another deep breath coming up.

Thigh Kick and Catch

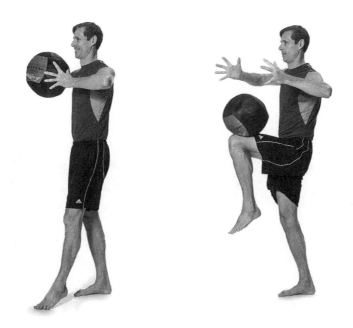

Start with most of your weight on one foot and the other foot lightly touching the floor in front of you. Grip the ball in front of your chest with your elbows pointed outward. Lift your knee straight up in front of you and drop the ball so that it bounces off your upper thigh. The ball should bounce up only a few inches. At the height of its bounce, grab the ball and lower your leg to the starting position.

Exhale with each kick. Complete all repetitions with one foot, then repeat with the other foot.

Crunch and Leg Extension

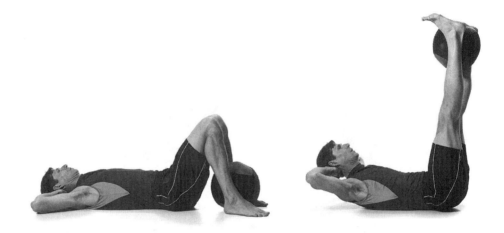

Lie on your back on the floor with your knees bent and your feet flat on the floor. Hold the ball between your feet, interlock your fingers behind your neck, and look straight up.

Keeping your elbows pointed out, do a crunch, lifting your upper body slowly off the floor. Simultaneously lift the ball up to the ceiling until your legs are fully extended or you can't straighten them any farther. Lower your upper body and the ball back to the floor at the same time. Breathe out while you're crunching up and again while you're lowering your body.

Good Morning

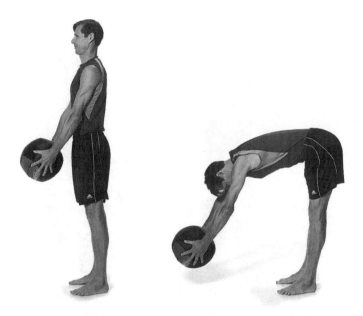

Begin with your feet parallel and less than shoulder-width apart. Bend over at your hips and hold the ball downward with your arms fully extended. Push the ball down to the floor near your feet, or as close to the floor as you can. Put most of your weight on the balls of your feet, but don't lift your heels from the floor.

Stand back most of the way up, but not completely upright, while keeping your arms fully extended toward the floor. Exhale as you move in each direction.

Mower

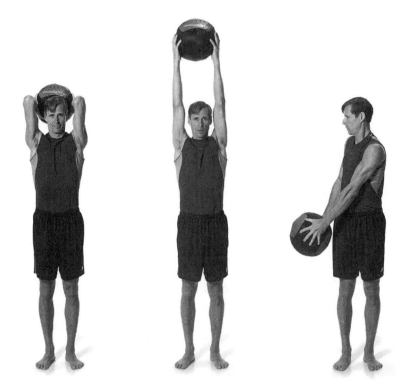

Begin in a parallel stance with your feet a few inches apart. Hold the ball in both hands behind the back of your neck. Try to keep your upper arms close to your ears. Reach up and extend your arms overhead into a soft lock, then bring the ball down to one side until your upper body has twisted toward that direction. Keep your arms fully extended and do not shrug your shoulders upward. Switch sides for each repetition. Exhale when you lower the ball and again when you lift your arms.

Using *Four Way Burn* for Peak Sports Performance

Soldier Walk

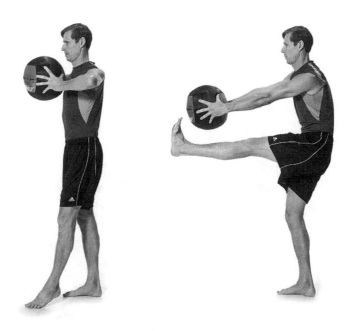

Begin with most of your weight on one foot and the other lightly touching the floor in front of you. Grip the ball in front of your chest with elbows pointed outward. Lift up your front leg while keeping it fully extended. At the same time, push the ball straight out and touch it to your lower shin when your leg reaches its maximum height. Exhale as you touch the ball to your shin.

Keeping your leg fully straightened, lower your foot back to the floor while you pull the ball back to your chest. Complete all repetitions on one side, then switch sides and repeat.

Straddle Squat and Reach

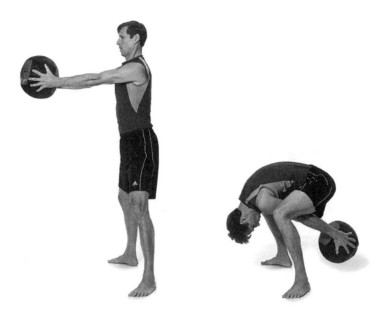

Begin with your feet parallel, but spaced very far apart. Your toes should be pointed outward. Press your big toes into the floor. Hold the ball at arm's length in front of your chest with both hands. Squat down, lean forward, and push the ball between your legs as far back as possible. This time, allow your entire back to become rounded as you push the ball so that you feel a good stretch in your lower back.

Exhale as you reach down, again as you hold the final position, and again as you stand up. Return to the starting point to finish the repetition.

Sit Up and Reach Overhead

Lie on the floor on your back with your knees bent and your feet flat on the floor. Hold the ball on your chest, firmly between both hands.

Sit up and simultaneously push the ball straight out in front of you, and then raise it over your head. Look straight ahead during the movement, and keep your heels anchored to the floor.

Lower yourself to the starting position to complete the repetition. Breathe out while you're sitting up and again when you're lowering yourself.

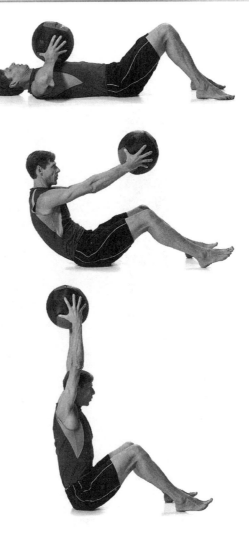

Good Morning with Side Twist

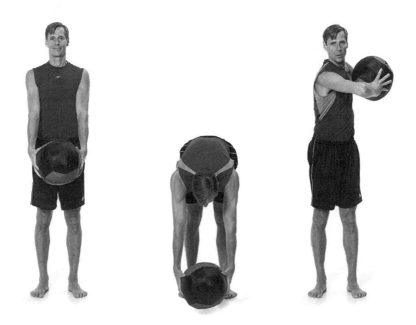

Begin with your feet parallel and closer than shoulder-width apart. At the starting position, hold the ball downward in front of your groin with your arms fully extended.

Lean straight down and touch the ball to the floor in front of your feet. Now stand up while bringing the ball to your chest, and fully twist your torso to one side. While twisting, make sure that your elbows don't drop below chest level. Return your torso so you're facing center to complete the repetition. Alternate between twisting left and right with each repetition.

Exhale as you bend down and as you twist.

Rocking Chair

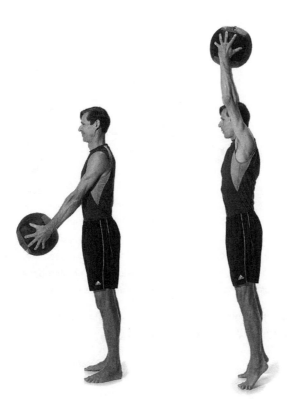

Begin with your feet in a parallel stance, spaced less than shoulder-width apart. Stand up straight and hold the ball so that it's hanging down in front of your groin, with your arms fully extended.

Rise up on your toes as you bring the ball straight overhead. Your arms should remain fully extended—never bending—at all times. If you can't bring the ball straight overhead, go as high as your flexibility allows. Now, lower the ball back to the starting position as you rock back onto your heels.

Breathe out as you rock on your feet in each direction.

Pecking Bird

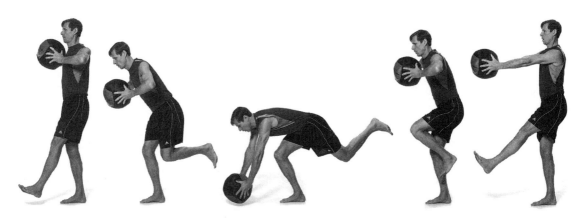

Stand on one foot, with your other leg extended in front of you and that foot raised a few inches off the floor. Hold the ball at chest level with your elbows out. Slowly lean forward, extend your arms, and touch the ball to the floor (or reach as far as you can). As you're leaning over, do a mini-squat on your standing leg, and bring your front leg back behind you, bending it at the knee. Straighten back up and push the ball out at chest level, simultaneously bringing your rear leg back out to the front.

Exhale four times—when you lean and squat down, stand back up, push out the ball, and pull it back to your chest. Complete all repetitions on that leg, then switch legs and repeat.

Using *Four Way Burn* for Peak Sports Performance

Atlas

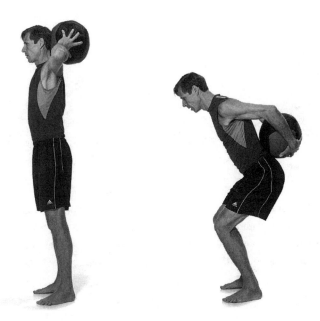

This exercise requires quick movements. Begin with your feet parallel and spaced just a few inches apart. Hold the ball against the back of your neck with both hands. Squat down and lean forward slightly, while keeping your back straight. Your head should be in line with your back, not craned back or forward.

Release the ball, then immediately move your hands so that you're reaching behind your lower back, and catch the ball when it arrives. The ball should roll smoothly between your shoulder blades and down your back, with no bouncing. To make the ball roll more slowly, lean farther forward.

When you catch the ball, bring it back around to your front, then resume the starting position. Exhale three times during the exercise: when the ball rolls down your spine, when you catch it, and when you place it behind your head.

Situp, Straight-Leg Raise, and Push

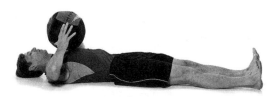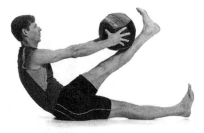

Lie on your back on the floor with your legs extended and feet flexed, holding the ball firmly between both hands against your chest. Sit up. While you are sitting up, simultaneously lift your left leg, keeping it fully extended. Then lean forward and push the ball out toward the toes on your left foot. You should feel a stretch behind your thighs and in your lower back. Lower yourself, then repeat. Breathe out as you sit up and again as you lower yourself. Complete all repetitions with one leg, then switch legs and repeat.

Using *Four Way Burn* for Peak Sports Performance

Triceps and Leg Extensions

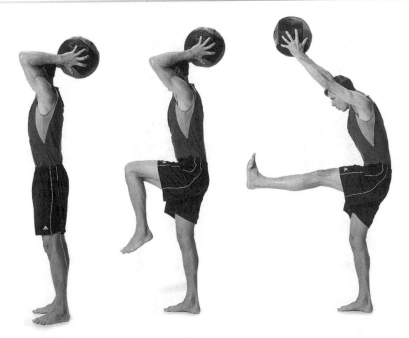

Begin in a parallel stance with your feet just a few inches apart. "Suck and tuck" your pelvis. Hold the ball with both hands behind the back of your neck, keeping your elbows close to your head. Lift one leg until your thigh is parallel with the floor, and extend your foot until your leg is straight. At the same time, bring the ball over your head and forward until your arms are fully extended at an upward angle toward the ceiling. Return to the starting position to complete the repetition. Alternate feet with each repetition. Exhale when you reach out with the ball and again when you pull it back.

Dough Kneading

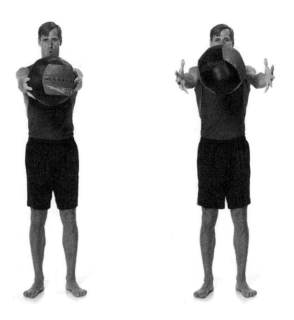

Begin with your feet in a narrow parallel stance. Hold the ball in front of your chest with your arms fully extended. All you're going to do is release the ball for a split second and grab it again, digging your fingertips and palms deeply into it. Quickly do this over and over, as if you're vigorously kneading a ball of dough. Focus on your "suck and tuck" posture. Exhale each time you catch the ball.

Crescent Reach

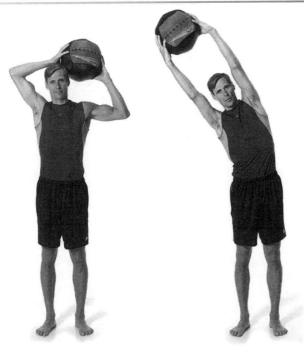

Begin in a parallel stance with a tall posture, your feet a few inches apart. Hold the ball firmly between your hands, above your left shoulder. Your elbows should point outward. Fully extend your arms upward and at an angle to the right while tilting your upper body to the right. Your arms should be alongside your head, not in front of it or behind it. Visualize your body shaped like a crescent moon.

Return your torso to center and lower the ball back to your shoulder, lowering your elbows down toward the floor, to complete the repetition. Exhale when you push the ball upward and again when you bring it back down. Complete the repetitions in one direction, then switch directions and repeat.

Knee Tuck and Push

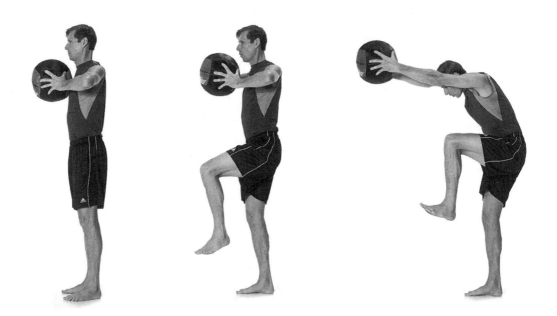

Begin in a parallel stance with your feet a few inches apart, while holding the ball in front of your chest with your elbows pointed outward.

Lift one thigh upward until it's higher than parallel with the floor, keeping your foot flexed. At the same time, lean your upper body forward and extend your arms in a soft lock so that the ball is held out from your body. It's okay to lower your head and hunch forward as you press the ball outward. Put more weight on the ball of the foot on which you're standing.

To complete the repetition, lower your foot and straighten that leg. Stand upright, and bring the ball back to your chest, keeping your elbows between chest and shoulder height and pulling your shoulder blades together. Exhale once as you push the ball away from you and again as you pull it back. Complete all repetitions on one side, then switch sides and repeat.

Situp, Knee Pull, and Chop

Lie on your back on the floor with your legs extended. Hold the ball firmly with both hands above your right shoulder and next to your right ear.

Sit up while pulling your left knee toward your chest. Tighten your abdominal muscles so that you pull your belly button inward.

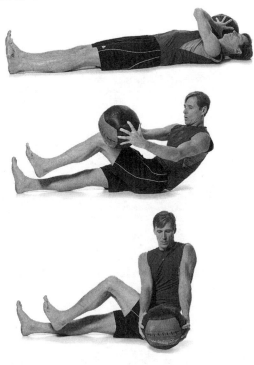

As you sit up, turn your upper body to the left side and "chop" the ball toward the floor. Both of your arms should become fully extended. In the final position, you should be sitting up with your right leg still on the floor, your left knee pulled close to your chest, and your upper body and both arms pointed out to the left.

Lower yourself to the floor to complete the repetition. Exhale when you sit up and again when you lower yourself down. Complete the repetitions in one direction, then switch directions and repeat.

Proper Bike Fit Can Reduce Injury Risk

Making sure that your bike is the correct size and that your body is properly positioned on it are critical factors for performing well, avoiding injuries, and having fun while bicycling. Here are some tips for keeping your bike maintained and adjusted.

- ▶ When you stand astride your bike, there should be an inch or two of space between the upper frame and your crotch.
- ▶ At the bottom of your pedal downstroke, your knee should remain slightly bent.
- ▶ Your saddle should either be level or have the front end angled very slightly upward.
- ▶ The height of the handlebars should be at least an inch or two below the top of the saddle.
- ▶ Consider working with a specialist at a bike shop to determine the best fit.

BICYCLING CONDITIONING CHART

WEEK 1

	Beginner	Intermediate	Advanced
Push and Pull	5 reps in all three directions	10 reps in all three directions	15 reps in all three directions
Saturn	10 reps each direction	15 reps each direction	20 reps each direction

Repeat the first two techniques for a second set, then move on to the next techniques.

	Beginner	Intermediate	Advanced
Squat and Push	10 reps	15 reps	20 reps
Thigh Kick and Catch	10 reps each leg	15 reps each leg	20 reps each leg
Crunch and Leg Extension	15 reps	20 reps	25 reps

Repeat the second group of techniques for a second set, then do the stretching/relaxation moves below (see pages 41 to 43).

Wedge

Lying Side Twist

Spread Eagle

WEEK 2

	Beginner	Intermediate	Advanced
Good Morning	10 reps	15 reps	20 reps
Mower	10 reps each side	12 reps each side	15 reps each side

Repeat the first two techniques for a second set, then move on to the next techniques.

	Beginner	Intermediate	Advanced
Soldier Walk	10 reps each leg	15 reps each leg	20 reps each leg
Straddle Squat and Reach	10 reps	15 reps	20 reps
Sit Up and Reach Overhead	10 reps	15 reps	20 reps

Repeat the second group of techniques for a second set, then do the stretching/relaxation moves below (see pages 41 to 43).

Wedge

Lying Side Twist

Spread Eagle

WEEK 3

	Beginner	Intermediate	Advanced
Good Morning with Side Twist	8 reps each side	10 reps each side	12 reps each side
Rocking Chair	10 reps	15 reps	20 reps

Repeat the first two techniques for a second set, then move on to the next techniques.

	Beginner	Intermediate	Advanced
Pecking Bird	8 reps each leg	10 reps each leg	12 reps each leg
Atlas	14 reps each direction	16 reps each direction	20 reps each direction
Situp, Straight-Leg Raise, and Push	10 reps each leg	12 reps each leg	15 reps each leg

Repeat the second group of techniques for a second set, then do the stretching/relaxation moves below (see pages 41 to 43).

Wedge

Lying Side Twist

Spread Eagle

WEEK 4

	Beginner	Intermediate	Advanced
Triceps and Leg Extensions	10 reps each leg	12 reps each leg	15 reps each leg
Dough Kneading	20 reps	25 reps	30 reps

Repeat the first two techniques for a second set, then move on to the next techniques.

	Beginner	Intermediate	Advanced
Crescent Reach	10 reps each side	12 reps each side	15 reps each side
Knee Tuck and Push	10 reps each leg	12 reps each leg	15 reps each leg
Situp, Knee Pull, and Chop	10 reps each side	12 reps each side	15 reps each side

Repeat the second group of techniques for a second set, then do the stretching/relaxation moves below (see pages 41 to 43).

Wedge

Lying Side Twist

Spread Eagle

12

GOLF: COMPLEX MOVES REQUIRE THOROUGH CONDITIONING

Hitting a golf ball accurately for 18 holes requires a full range of your body's capabilities. You need dynamic balance—which means holding your body in the right position while it moves. You need coordination, flexibility, and strength. And you need the stamina to maintain your power and form for the entire 18 holes.

All your body parts must work together fluidly with each swing. More than 35 major muscle groups are involved in hitting a golf ball. Your nervous system must activate them in the proper sequence in order to achieve a fluid and effective swing with a controlled speed and tempo.

Although your whole body is involved in a golf swing, the various parts and muscle groups play different roles throughout the stroke:

- ▶ Your leg muscles generate most of the golf swing's power and are important for a supportive and solid foundation.
- ▶ Your core muscles—the abdomen, waist, and lower back—are responsible for the energy transfer from your legs to your torso. These muscles are responsible for swing acceleration.
- ▶ Your upper torso—including your chest, lats (along the sides of your back), and shoulders—produces the actual swinging action and plays a big role in generating club head speed. Your entire arms, including your biceps and triceps, forearms, wrists, hands, and fingers, control the accuracy of the club head on impact with the golf ball.

The *Four Way Burn* program is an ideal way to improve all the fitness elements that you use on the golf course. You will build strength proportionately in your upper and lower body, without making your muscles tight or bulky. You will proportionately strengthen opposing muscles—such as your biceps and triceps—to reduce your risk of overuse injuries. Plus, you will improve the resilience of your tendons and ligaments, thus protecting easily injured parts such as your rotator cuffs, elbows, wrists, lower back, and knees.

At the same time, you'll build other skills that are equally important. You'll reinforce proper stance and body mechanics, which reduces fatigue and improves your awareness of proper body positioning on the course. And by squeezing and handling the ball, you'll improve your control over the golf club.

Golf relies as much on the mind as on the body, and my training method is specifically designed to make the two work better together. Each technique requires your mind and body to constantly provide feedback to each other, back and forth. The muscles, nervous system, and mind all work in harmony.

You're making a lot of improvements all at one time, which means you don't have to spend hours a week in the gym . . . which means more hours you can spend out on the golf course!

The golf conditioning program consists of four cycles, each containing six conditioning techniques and three relaxation/stretching techniques. Do one set of each of the first three techniques, then go through them again for a second set. Move on to the second three techniques, and do a set of each, then repeat for the second set. Then move on to the relaxation/ stretching techniques. The relaxation stretches are also good for after you return home from a golf game.

Do two sessions a week on days that you're not playing golf. Spend 25 to 30 minutes on each session.

During times when you're not playing golf at all, return to doing the original *Four Way Burn* program described earlier in the book.

Push and Pull

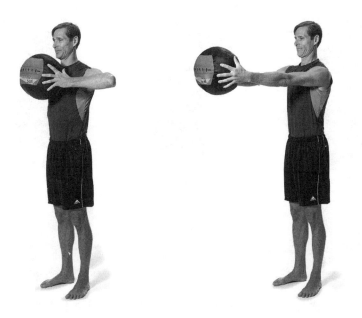

Begin in a parallel stance, with your feet side by side and spaced shoulder-width apart.

At the beginning of the motion, start by holding the ball at your chest, with your elbows pointed out to the sides. Push the ball out until your arms are fully extended in a "soft lock." On the first third of the repetitions, push the ball straight out. On the next third of the repetitions, push it out diagonally to your left. On the final third of the repetitions, push it out diagonally to your right. While pushing out at an angle, twist your upper body toward that particular side. Draw the ball back to your chest, and repeat.

Breathe out as you push the ball away from you, inhale, and breathe out again as you pull the ball toward you.

Saturn

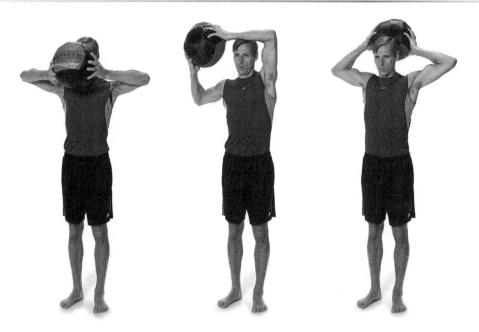

Stand in a parallel stance with your feet less than shoulder-width apart. Grip the ball in both hands in front of your face, with your elbows pointed outward. Now, rotate the ball around your head in a circle. As it travels around your head, keep your elbows pointed outward. Breathe out for half of the circle around your head, and breathe in for the other half.

Do the recommended number of repetitions, then switch directions and repeat for the same number. All the repetitions in both directions equal one set.

Side Twist

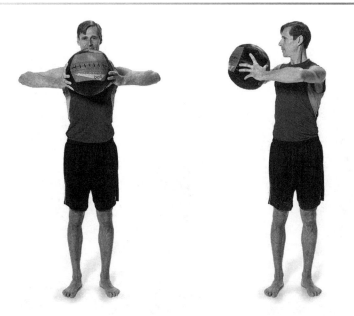

Begin with your feet in a parallel stance, your hands holding the ball in front of your chest and your elbows pointing out to the sides. Begin twisting your torso from side to side, using the core muscles around your abdomen and lower back to provide movement. You should only be twisting your upper body—not twisting at the knees. Each repetition requires you to fully twist one way, then the other.

Exhale one long breath as you move in each direction.

Hula Hoop

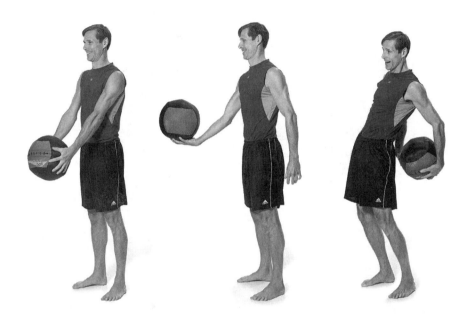

Begin with your feet parallel and close together. Grip the ball firmly between both hands and hold it in front of your abdomen. Start rotating the ball around your body, scooping it up from hand to hand as it passes your midsection and back. Much like a hula hoop, it should travel smoothly around and around your body.

Rotate your hips as the ball passes around your body. Breathe out as the ball passes behind your back and again when it goes across your front. When you have completed all your repetitions in one direction, repeat, moving the ball in the opposite direction.

Squat and Push

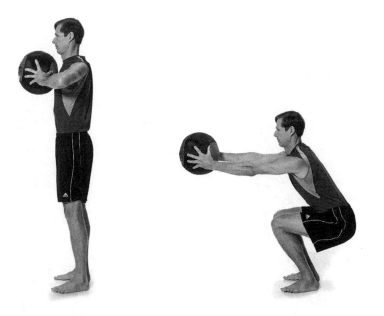

Begin in a parallel stance. Start by holding the ball in front of your chest with your elbows pointed outward. Now, squat down. As you squat, fully extend the ball away from you until your arms are straightened in a soft lock. Look straight ahead at all times.

As you squat, keep your feet flat—don't rise up on your toes. As you stand up, simultaneously pull the ball back to your chest and squeeze your shoulder blades together. Take in one deep breath going down, exhale, and take in another deep breath coming up.

Soldier Walk

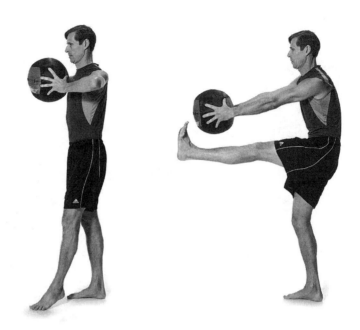

Begin with most of your weight on one foot and the other foot lightly touching the floor in front of you. Grip the ball in front of your chest, with your elbows pointed outward. Lift your front leg while keeping it fully extended. At the same time, push the ball straight out and touch it to your lower shin when your leg reaches its maximum height. Exhale as you touch the ball to your shin.

Keeping your leg fully straightened, lower your foot back to the floor while you pull the ball back to your chest. Complete all repetitions with one foot, and switch legs and repeat.

Using Four Way Burn for Peak Sports Performance

Good Morning

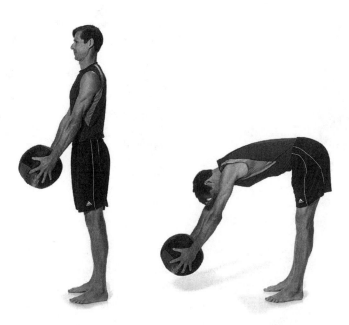

Begin with your feet parallel and less than shoulder-width apart. Bend over at your hips and hold the ball downward with your arms fully extended. Push the ball down to the floor near your feet, or as close to the floor as you can. Put most of your weight on the balls of your feet, but don't lift your heels from the floor.

Stand back most of the way up, but not completely upright, while keeping your arms fully extended toward the floor. Exhale as you move in each direction.

Discus

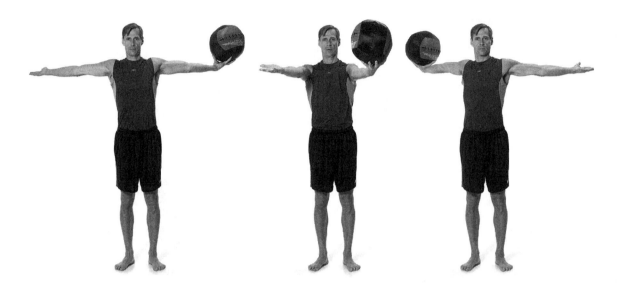

Stand in a parallel stance, with your feet closer than shoulder-width apart. Hold the ball in one hand and bring your arm out to your side, keeping your elbow in a soft lock and your arm fully extended the entire time. At the same time, bring your other arm out to your other side. Use the full range of motion as you move your arms out to the sides.

Now, bring both hands back in front of you—keeping your arms fully extended—and pass the ball to your other hand. Bring your arms back out to your sides. Keep repeating and passing the ball from hand to hand. Exhale while reaching out in each direction.

The Coil

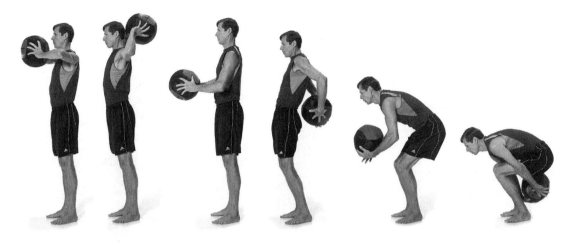

To begin, start in the Saturn position (see page 32). Move the ball around your head, then smoothly lower it and pass it around your midsection. As the ball comes back around to your abdomen, squat down and pass it behind your legs and back in front of you. Now, keep moving the ball up and around your body in a Hula Hoop (see page 36) and a Saturn until it ends in front of your face. Going all the way down and all the way up is one repetition. Exhale as the ball passes in front of you each time. Complete all repetitions in one direction, then switch directions and repeat.

Golfer Swing

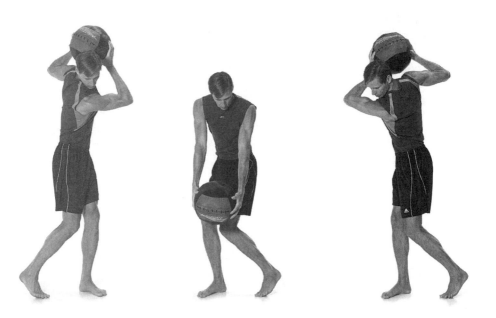

Begin with your feet positioned parallel and less than shoulder-width apart. Extend your arms and hold the ball in front of your groin. Bring the ball with both hands up to one shoulder, as if you're setting up to swing a golf club. Just before you make this motion, start pivoting your feet so that they point toward the direction the ball is traveling. Your entire body will be pivoting as you bring the ball above your shoulder. At the highest point, bend both elbows.

When you reach your highest point and have finished the upward motion, pivot your feet the other way and move the ball back down, across your groin and up to your other shoulder. Your arms and the ball will look like a pendulum swinging down and up from shoulder to shoulder, as your feet pivot back and forth. Exhale forcefully with each swing. Complete all the repetitions on one side, then switch sides and repeat.

Statue of Liberty

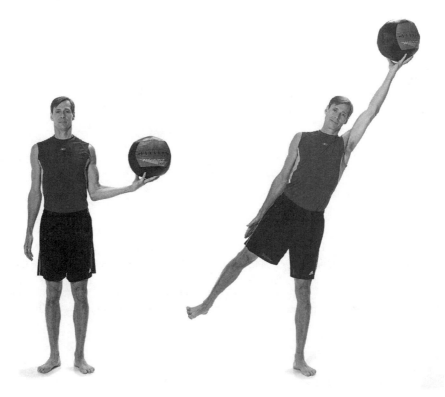

Begin with your feet parallel and just a few inches apart. Hold the ball in one hand, with your arm at your side and bent at a 90-degree angle.

Slowly extend the arm with the ball, reaching up and out over your shoulder as you lift your opposite leg up and out to the side, as shown. Return your arm and your leg to their starting point to complete the repetition. Complete all the repetitions on one side, then switch sides and repeat.

Breathe out when your arms and legs come together, and again when they move apart.

Spider Walk

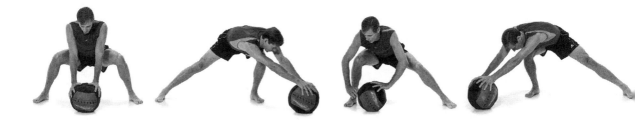

Begin with your feet in a parallel stance but spaced more than shoulder-width apart. Set the ball on the floor so that you're straddling it, and place both hands on the ball. Bend your knees and lower your buttocks until your thighs are parallel to the floor, and dig into the floor with your big toes.

With both hands, roll the ball out to the left away from you as far as you can go. Roll it back to the center, then out to the right to complete one repetition. Take two breaths while rolling the ball in each direction.

Behind-the-Leg Pass

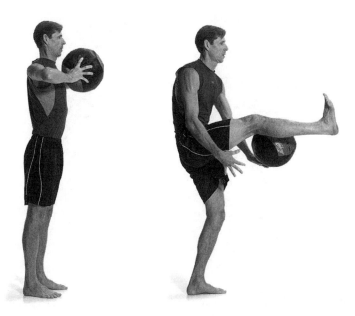

Begin with your feet parallel and spaced a few inches apart. Hold the ball in front of your chest with your elbows pointed outward.

Lift your leg straight up and pass the ball under your leg. The ball should travel to the outside of your thigh, under, and back up past your inner thigh, and end in both hands above your leg again. Lower your leg back to the starting position to complete the repetition. Do this in one smooth motion—imagine a basketball player passing the ball under his leg.

Exhale when you pass the ball under your leg. Complete all the repetitions with one leg, then repeat with the other.

Twist and Sweep

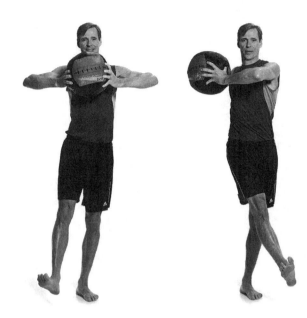

Start by standing on your left foot, with your right foot lifted a few inches in front of you. Hold the ball in front of your chest with your elbows pointing outward. Twist your upper chest (and the ball) to the right while sweeping your right foot to the left. Your pelvis should stay stationary and your abdominals and lower back should control the motion—but only your chest and leg should move.

During this motion, your leg should remain straight and your foot should stay pointed forward. Imagine putting a golf ball with your instep, then the outer edge of your foot, as your foot sweeps from side to side. Breathe out as you twist in either direction. Complete all repetitions on one side, then switch sides.

Carioca Loop

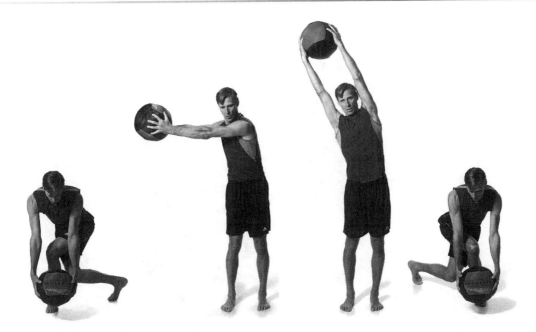

Begin by squatting down with most of your weight on your left leg, and your right foot touching the floor behind you and out to your left. Both knees should be bent and your right foot should be resting on the ball of your foot. Lean forward, fully extend your arms, and let the ball hang to your left knee.

Keeping your arms fully extended, bring the ball in a wide circle toward the right, then overhead, while at the same time stepping up with your back foot into a parallel stance. You should reach this stance just as the ball reaches the point straight overhead. Continue moving the ball in a circle toward the left and down as you step behind with your left foot. You will end up with most of your weight on your right leg, with your left leg behind you and out to your right, and your arms fully extended and holding the ball just below your right knee. This is the mirror opposite of how you started.

Exhale while you're lifting and lowering the ball. Return to the starting position for your next rep. Complete all repetitions in this direction, then switch directions and repeat.

Straddle Squat and Reach

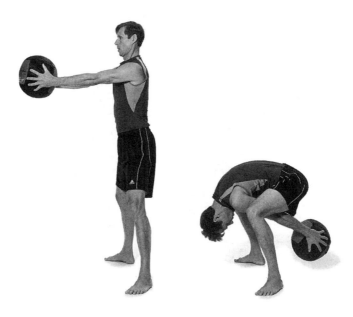

Begin with your feet parallel, but spaced very far apart. Your toes should point outward. Press your big toes into the floor. Hold the ball at arm's length in front of your chest with both hands. Squat down, lean forward, and push the ball between your legs as far back as possible. This time, allow your entire back to become rounded as you push the ball so you feel a good stretch in your lower back.

Exhale as you reach down, again as you hold the final position, and again as you stand up. Return to the starting point to finish the repetition.

Around the World

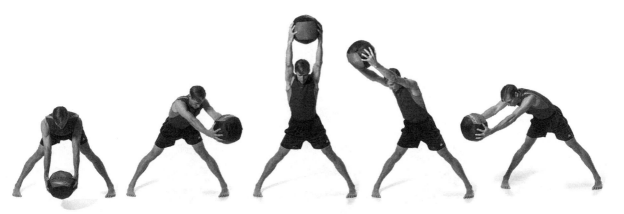

Begin with your feet in a parallel stance, spaced farther than shoulder-width apart. Keep your legs straight, with your toes pointed inward and pressed into the floor.

Lean forward deeply and hold the ball toward the floor in both hands, with your arms fully extended. Reaching out as far as you can, move the ball out to your left and up until it's overhead, and on to your right and back down to the starting point. As you reach the high point of this circle, stretch yourself up as tall as you can. Keep your arms and legs straight as you make the circle.

Exhale as your hands travel past each quarter of the circle. Finish all repetitions in one direction, then switch directions.

Mower

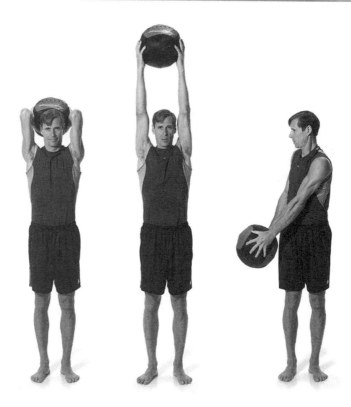

Begin in a parallel stance with your feet a few inches apart. Hold the ball in both hands behind the back of your neck. Try to keep your upper arms close to your ears. Reach up and extend your arms overhead into a soft lock, then bring the ball down to one side until your upper body has twisted toward that direction. Keep your arms fully extended and do not shrug your shoulders upward. Switch sides for each repetition.

Exhale when you lower the ball and again when you lift your arms.

Using *Four Way Burn* for Peak Sports Performance

Split Stand Reach to Toes

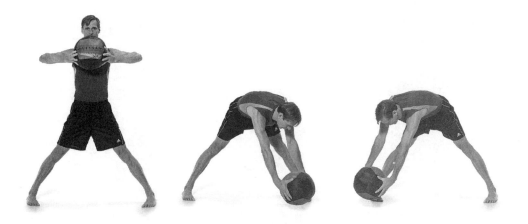

Begin in a very wide parallel stance with your legs straight and your toes pointed inward. Hold the ball to your chest with your elbows pointed outward.

Lean forward and, with your arms fully extended, try to touch one foot with the ball, or reach out even farther. Stand back up and pull the ball to your chest to complete the repetition. Breathe out when you reach down and again when you lift yourself up. Complete all the repetitions on one side, then switch sides and repeat.

Good Morning with Side Twist

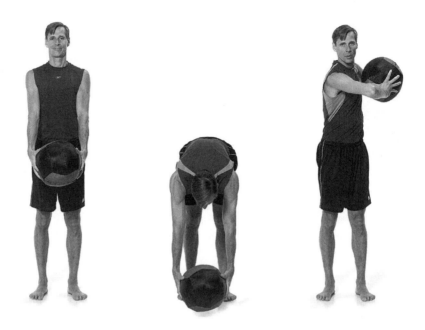

Begin with your feet parallel and closer than shoulder-width apart. At the starting position, hold the ball downward in front of your groin with your arms fully extended.

Lean straight down and touch the ball to the floor in front of your feet. Now stand up while bringing the ball to your chest, and fully twist your torso to one side. While twisting, make sure your elbows don't drop below chest level. Return your torso so you're facing center to complete the repetition. Alternate between twisting left and right with each repetition.

Exhale as you bend down and as you twist.

Race Car Driver

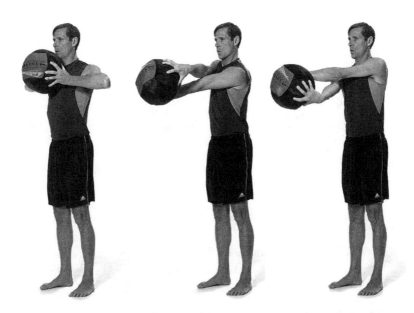

Begin in a parallel stance with your feet a few inches apart. Stand tall. Hold the ball between both hands at your chest. Extend your arms in a soft lock in front of your chest. Your hands should be placed at the left and right sides of the ball. Counter the weight you are holding by "sucking and tucking" your pelvis. This will prevent you from arching your back.

Now, twist the ball between your hands as if you're turning a steering wheel. Your arms may touch if you twist the ball far enough, but twist only as far as is comfortable. When you have twisted as far as you can in one direction, twist to the other direction to complete one repetition. Exhale with each rotation.

Figure Eight Walk

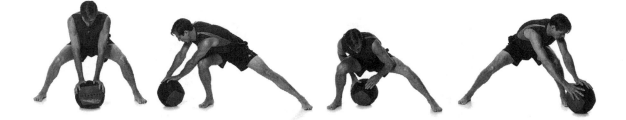

Begin in a wide parallel stance, with your feet spaced as far apart as you can comfortably get them. Lean forward and place the ball on the floor in front of you. Pushing the ball with both hands, roll it around and between your legs so that its path forms a figure eight around your feet. Shift your upper body as you move the ball so that your chest stays pointed at the ball throughout its movement. Push your body toward the direction in which you are passing the ball, to improve your reach.

Take four breaths for each figure eight pass. Return to the starting point as you begin your next rep. After completing all repetitions in this direction, rotate the ball in the opposite direction and repeat.

Using *Four Way Burn* for Peak Sports Performance

Front-Arm Raise with Leg Abduction

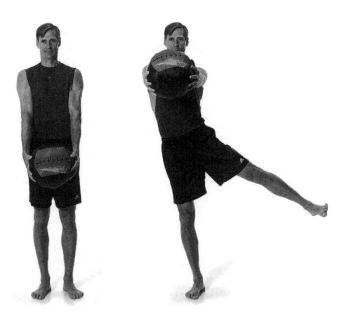

Stand in a parallel stance with your feet shoulder-width apart. Hold the ball in both hands with a strong grip and your arms fully extended so that the ball is in front of your groin. Lift one leg out to the side while lifting the ball upward until your arms are parallel to the floor, keeping your arms and legs fully extended. To complete the repetition, lower your arms to the starting position and lower your foot until your heels touch.

Exhale when lifting the ball and again when lowering it. Complete all of the repetitions, then switch sides and repeat.

Dough Kneading

Begin with your feet in a narrow parallel stance. Hold the ball in front of your chest with your arms fully extended. All you're going to do is release the ball for a split second and grab it again, digging your fingertips and palms deeply into it. Quickly do this over and over, as if you're vigorously kneading a ball of dough. Focus on your "suck and tuck" posture. Exhale each time you catch the ball.

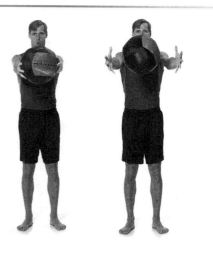

Richard Madris

"I can do things today that I might not have been able to do when I was 40," says Richard Madris, a 62-year-old real estate investor and former garment manufacturer.

Richard has been a client for about 20 years. We've incorporated into his workouts different fitness developments that were worth keeping and passed over the trends and novelties that weren't. But the *Four Way Burn* techniques with a weighted ball have remained a central part of his sessions.

"The Performance Ball has been a very strong influence on my workout sessions," Richard says. "They're exciting, invigorating, new, and fun. I call Ralf 'Dr. Frankenstein' . . . I say, 'have you been working in your lab creating new uses for your Performance Ball?'

"One thing about working out with Ralf is it's never boring because he always works out something innovative for me. He's very dedicated to the success of helping people rehabilitate or helping people just feel generally good about themselves," he says.

"Once I was walking on a slope on some wet grass, and I fell with my right arm back behind me. I felt like I'd pulled my arm, and I couldn't even lift a 2-pound weight. I told Ralf what happened. We spent 2 years rehabbing it—incorporating the workout to be specific to my shoulder injury, but not neglecting the rest of my body. Today the shoulder is stronger and has more flexibility and range of motion," he says. "It's helped me with my golf game tremendously."

GOLF CONDITIONING CHART

CYCLE ONE (2 WEEKS)	CYCLE TWO (2 WEEKS)	CYCLE THREE (2 WEEKS)	CYCLE FOUR (2 WEEKS)
Push and Pull 5 reps in each direction	**Good Morning** 15 reps in each direction	**Behind-the-Leg Pass** 5 reps in each direction with each leg (20 total)	**Split Stand Reach to Toes** 10 reps each side
Saturn 10 reps in each direction	**Discus** 15 reps each arm	**Twist and Sweep** 15 reps each side	**Good Morning with Side Twist** 10 reps each side
Side Twist 15 reps in each direction	**The Coil** 5 reps in each direction	**Carioca Loop** 10 reps each side	**Race Car Driver** 15 reps each side
Repeat the first three exercises for a second set, then move to the next three.			
Hula Hoop 15 reps in each direction	**Golfer Swing** 20 reps in each direction	**Straddle Squat and Reach** 15 reps	**Figure Eight Walk** 10 reps each side
Squat and Push 15 reps	**Statue of Liberty** 10 reps each side	**Around the World** 5 reps in each direction	**Front-Arm Raise with Leg Abduction** 10 reps each side
Soldier Walk 10 reps each leg	**Spider Walk** 10 reps each side	**Mower** 10 reps each side	**Dough Kneading** 30 reps
Repeat the second three exercises for a second set, then move to the relaxation/stretching techniques below. (See pages 41 to 43.)			
Wedge	Wedge	Wedge	Wedge
Lying Side Twist	Lying Side Twist	Lying Side Twist	Lying Side Twist
Spread Eagle	Spread Eagle	Spread Eagle	Spread Eagle

13

INCREASE CONTROL AND POWER ON THE TENNIS COURT

One of my jobs as a fitness professional during the 1980s was working at Ivan Lendl's tennis training center. At the time, Lendl was the top-ranked player in the world, and his center attracted many other leading players and teaching professionals. I led group fitness classes and had fun playing tennis against some *very* good opponents.

In those days, improving one's fitness specifically for the game of tennis was still in its infancy, and I introduced it at Lendl's camp. Simply playing the game over and over doesn't provide proper conditioning—you must improve your strength, flexibility, and coordination *off* the court, too.

Nowadays, it's common for professional tennis players to work with strength and conditioning coaches as part of their training regimens, to become better prepared for their games. But even casual players should follow a program to perform better in the physical challenges they're going to face.

The quick, complex movements of the *Four Way Burn* program are great preparation for tennis. When you become physically fatigued during the game, your balance, coordination, quickness, agility, strength, and timing all become compromised. By training hard off the court, you may be able to go longer than your opponent without tiring.

In addition, the conditioning program in this chapter will give you excellent mobility. Lunging, twisting, turning, reaching, and leaning while moving are all part of the tennis game. Without good flexibility, your movements will be limited and your risk of injury will increase. In the technique descriptions, I've included a list of tennis-specific benefits for each movement.

CONDITION YOUR BODY TO MEET THE DEMANDS OF THE GAME

Here's an overview of the specific challenges your body parts face during a game of tennis.

Your fingers, hands, and arms. A tennis ball can exceed 100 miles per hour, and tennis racket technology is constantly being improved to allow you to hit the ball more powerfully and accurately. However, your fingers, hands, wrists, and arms need to be strong to absorb and control the energy from your racket. Most recreational players aren't aware that they need a higher level of conditioning to make use of new rackets. But without enough strength, even an expensive racket will be ineffective.

As you're working through the *Four Way Burn* tennis techniques, be sure to keep a tight grip on the ball and move your wrists and elbows through their full range of motion. Without proper strength and conditioning in your hands and arms, your strokes will quickly become sluggish and irregular.

Your shoulders. Strong shoulders are important for powerful volleys, serves, and returns. However, without proper flexibility, you will lose your valuable range of motion needed to swing the racket. And without good mobility, you will be prone to injury from sprains or strains. In addition, your upper back muscles must be sufficiently strong to counter the force created in the front of your body and to balance out your rear shoulder girdle.

Too much emphasis in the front of your body (which is where the action is in tennis) without strengthening your upper back will eventually cause injuries in your neck, shoulders, or rotator cuffs.

Your abdominal and lower back muscles. These muscles work as a team to twist and turn your body in preparation for a lob, smash, drop shot, or groundstroke. Without the strength of these core muscles, you're less able to transfer energy between your upper and lower body.

In addition, the abdominal and back muscles also stabilize the torso and hold it motionless when necessary. Because these muscles need to work as a team to prevent overuse and neglect, you need to train and condition them together.

Your hips. Running from side to side on the baseline, and forward to the net and back, requires solid hip support. Your buttocks, hip flexors, groin muscles, and hamstrings are all needed to accelerate, change directions quickly, and leap so you can react quickly to your opponent's strokes. Common injuries in the groin and hamstrings can be prevented with stronger support in and around the hips.

Your legs. If your legs aren't strong, you have less freedom to move about the court. Eventually you'll either become sluggish and fatigued before the match is over, or you'll get hurt.

Also, you need strength and flexibility to lunge and squat low to the ground. If you can't bend your hips and legs, your lower back will have to do extra work—work it was not designed to do.

Fast stops and quick changes compromise the stability of your knees. Dynamic balancing as you perform the techniques in my program will help to stabilize and strengthen your knees.

Strengthening your hamstrings, as well as muscles in the quadriceps of your thighs called the vastus medialis obliques, or VMOs, will also help protect your joints by strengthening a supportive ligament in the knee called the ACL.

Your ankles and feet. Your entire body weight is constantly placed on each foot while you play tennis, so both feet need to be extra-strong to support your weight. In addition, stability throughout the foot is key for holding your body motionless during various strokes.

Due to the constant lunging—mainly diagonally and sideways—the tennis player's foot becomes stronger on the outside but weaker on the inside. As a result, eversion ankle strains (rolling on the outside of the foot) are often seen in tennis, but they're avoidable. To correctly balance your feet for playing, you need stability training that supports the specific moves your feet make on the tennis court.

THE *FOUR WAY BURN* TENNIS PROGRAM

I've designed this program with the intention that you'll do it before you start playing tennis regularly to get your body ready for the sport. (For instance, if you begin playing tennis during the summer, start this program in the late spring.)

The program is broken into three 2-week cycles, each containing five techniques and another three stretching/relaxation movements.

During each session, do the first two techniques, performing one set of each, then go through them again, performing a second set. Then do a set of each of the next three techniques, then another set of them. End the session with the three movements that relax and stretch your muscles.

During the tennis season, select any five of these techniques of your choosing and do them three times a week on days when you're not playing any tennis matches.

Pull and Chop

Benefits: Conditions your rotator cuff and shoulders and strengthens your core, back, and trunk muscles to meet the high power demands of serving.

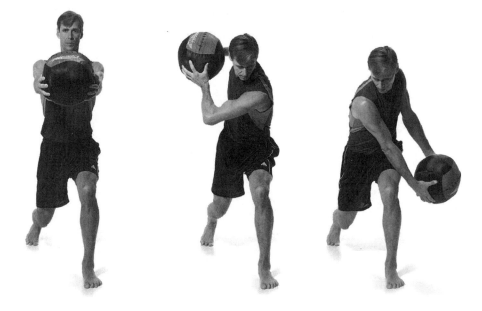

Stand in a split stance with your left foot forward and your body weight evenly distributed over both feet. Hold the ball with a firm grip and your arms fully extended. Inhale deeply. While exhaling, bend your arms and pull the ball over your right shoulder while simultaneously rotating your upper body in the same direction.

Now "chop" the ball down diagonally in a quick motion. While chopping, rotate your upper body to the left, lean forward, bend your knees and hips, and breathe forcefully out. Repeat this technique rhythmically for the desired number of repetitions, then switch your leg position and perform the same exercise in the opposite direction.

Rocking Chair

Benefits: Improves shoulder mobility, increases arm strength for
a better serve, and improves ankle stabilization for a more powerful reach.

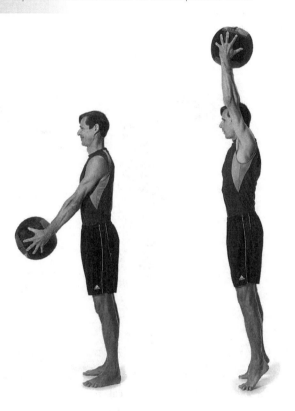

Begin with your feet in a parallel stance, spaced less than shoulder-width apart. Stand up straight and hold the ball so that it's hanging down in front of your groin with your arms fully extended.

Rise up on your toes as you bring the ball straight overhead. Your arms should remain fully extended—never bending—at all times. If you can't bring the ball straight overhead, go as high as your flexibility allows. Now lower the ball back to the starting position as you rock back onto your heels. Breathe out as you rock on your feet in each direction.

Make sure to keep your abdominal muscles and buttocks tight and firm.

Race Car Driver

Benefits: Strengthens your hands, arms, shoulders, and chest muscles; helps prevent tennis elbow; improves foot speed and strengthens your ankles; improves hand-eye and foot-eye coordination; and improves your stamina.

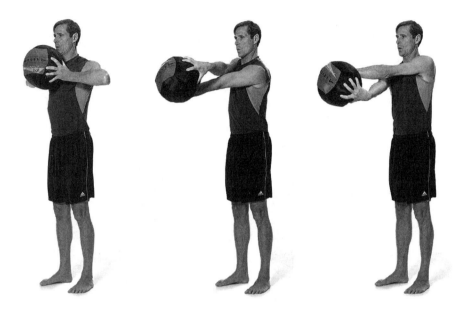

Begin in a parallel stance with your feet a few inches apart. Stand tall. Hold the ball between both hands at your chest. Extend your arms in a soft lock in front of your chest. Your hands should be placed at the left and right sides of the ball. Counter the weight you are holding by "sucking and tucking" your pelvis. This will prevent you from arching your back.

Now, twist the ball between your hands as if you're turning a steering wheel. Your arms may touch if you twist the ball far enough, but only twist as far as is comfortable. When you have twisted as far as you can in one direction, twist to the other direction to complete one repetition. Exhale with each rotation.

Triple Jump, Forward Lunge, and Side Twist

Benefits: Creates faster feet and stronger ankles and hip, abdominal, back, and leg muscles; improves stride length; and improves preparation for forehand and backhand shots.

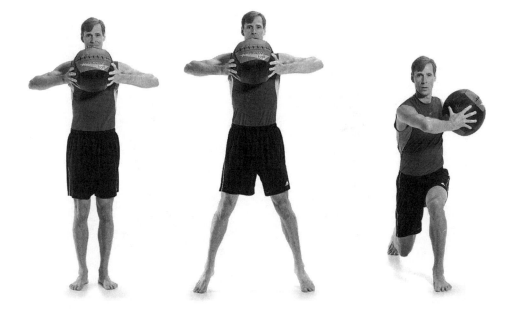

Stand up straight with your feet together, and hold the ball at chest height. Do three jumping jack motions with your legs, then immediately lunge forward with your left leg and twist your upper body to the left while holding the ball at chest height. Exhale while twisting. Return to the starting position. Complete all repetitions on one side, then switch sides and repeat.

Alternating Diagonal Lunge and Reach

Benefits: Strengthens and stretches your groin and inner thigh muscles; creates a longer and more powerful stride to cover the court; strengthens shoulders, elbows, and rotator cuffs; improves quickness and recovery; and encourages better hand-eye coordination and better spatial awareness.

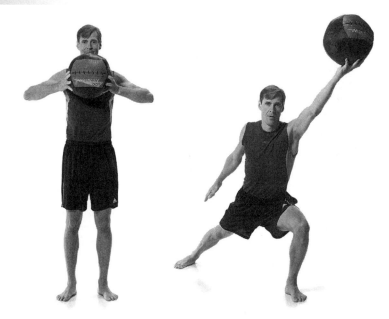

Stand upright with your feet together in a parallel stance while you balance on the balls of your feet. Hold the ball at chest level in both hands.

Inhale deeply. Exhale and lunge diagonally to the left with your left foot. As you do so, take the ball in your left hand and extend your left hand out diagonally to the left until your arm is fully extended. This would be a similar motion to starting with the racket in both hands, transferring it to your left hand, and lunging out to return a ball. Lean and reach as far as you can. Inhale and quickly come back to the starting position. Repeat toward the other side, alternating for the desired number of repetitions.

Using *Four Way Burn* for Peak Sports Performance

CYCLE TWO

Knead and Jump

Benefits: Strengthens your chest, shoulders, and elbow muscles; strengthens wrists and fingers; improves balance and leg power; and reduces your vulnerability to ankle, knee, and hip injuries.

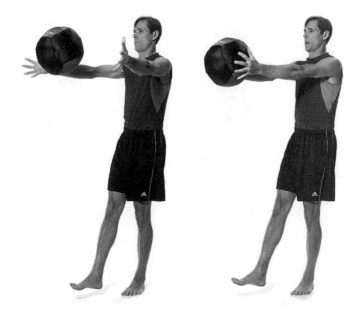

Stand on one leg and jump up and down. While jumping, fully extend both arms at chest level and alternately release and squeeze the ball rhythmically as if you were kneading bread dough. Keep your abdominal muscles tight and maintain good balance. Continue for 15 seconds, rest a moment, and repeat with the other leg.

Triple Jump, Back Lunge, and Side Twist

Benefits: Improves foot speed; allows you to make quicker directional changes while maintaining dynamic balance; improves strength of inner thigh and groin muscles; and develops functionally stronger core muscles and gluteal and leg muscles, which leads to better control in preparing the racket for the stroke.

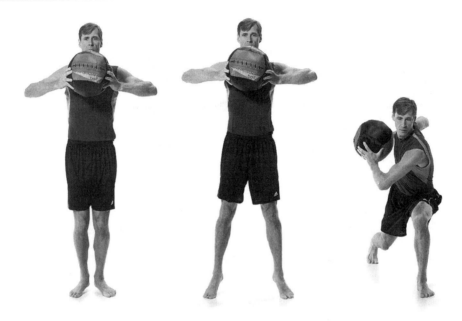

Balance yourself on the balls of your feet, with your feet in a parallel stance and close together, and hold the ball firmly at chest height with your elbows pointed out. Do three quick jumping jacks with your feet— spreading your feet to a little wider than shoulder-width—then extend your right leg behind you in a lunge position and twist your upper body to the right side. Exhale while lunging back and returning to the starting position. Complete all repetitions on one side, then change sides and repeat.

Using Four Way Burn for Peak Sports Performance

Squat and Racket Reach

Benefits: Strengthens your knees, hips, quadriceps, lower back, and abdominal muscles and creates better hand-eye coordination. It's also a great practice drill that allows you to drop low to the ground without compromising your lower back.

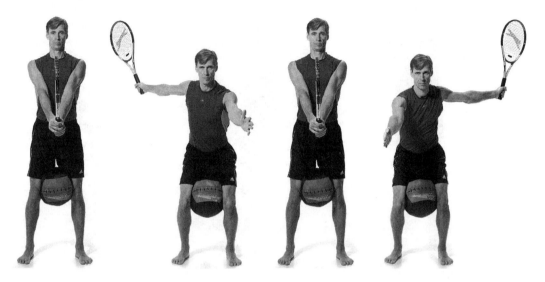

Hold the ball between your knees and thighs, and hold your racket in both hands. Squat down, maintaining a straight back, and transfer the racket to your right hand. Extend your right arm out as far to the right as possible while exhaling. Inhale, then exhale and stand upright. Repeat the same sequence to the left. Remember to keep your heels on the floor and your back flat and straight while squatting.

Jump and Twist

Benefits: Strengthens your ankles, knees, and hips; adds height to your vertical leap; reinforces core muscles; and adds power to your backhand and forehand.

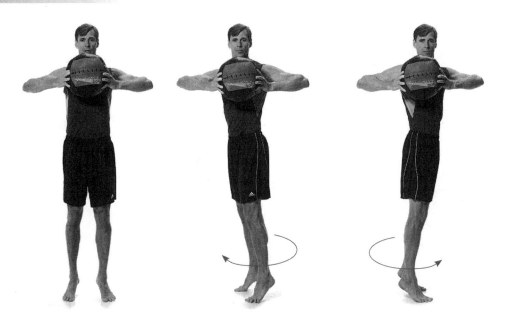

Hold the ball with a firm grip at chest level. Keeping your legs together, bounce up and down and pivot back and forth on the balls of your feet. As you're bouncing, twist your hips and feet to one direction while your upper body and arms turn to the other side. With each bounce, exhale.

Side Shuffle, Drop, Clap, and Catch

Benefits: Strengthens your hips, legs, and ankles specifically for court sports; improves your stamina, quickness, and reaction time; sharpens your hand-eye coordination; increases your mental focus; and strengthens your lower back.

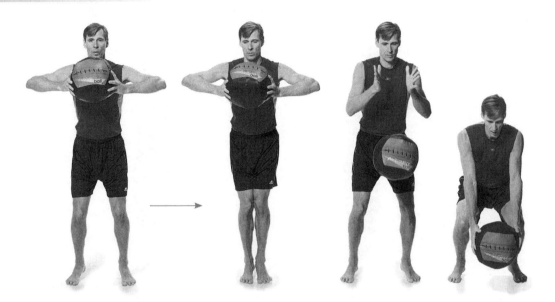

Hold the ball in your hands at chest height. Spread your feet about 2 inches wider than shoulder-width, and balance yourself on the balls of your feet.

Lean forward at the hips, keeping your back straight. Shuffle with exaggerated steps five times to one side (breathe out with each step), then drop the ball from chest level to the floor. Quickly clap your hands twice and catch the ball after one bounce. Your feet, knees, and hips should point forward the entire time. Shuffle to the opposite side five steps and repeat the technique.

Quick Feet Push and Pull

Benefits: Makes your feet faster; adds power to your upper body and core muscles; and improves your anaerobic energy system.

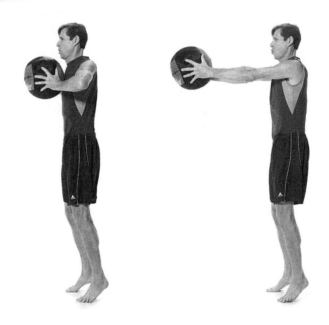

Hold the ball firmly at chest level with your elbows pointed outward. Keep your feet shoulder-width apart and balance on the balls of your feet. For the next 15 seconds, rapidly shuffle your feet so that your body weight goes back and forth between your feet. It's a little like tap dancing. At the same time, simulate tossing the ball to someone in front of you, but don't let go of the ball. Breathe forcefully and rhythmically.

Straight-Arm Toss, Hand Clap, and Catch

Benefits: Strengthens your arms, hands, and wrists to control the high velocity of an incoming serve; prevents tennis elbow (tendinitis); improves shoulder mobility; and improves reaction time, hand-eye coordination, and timing.

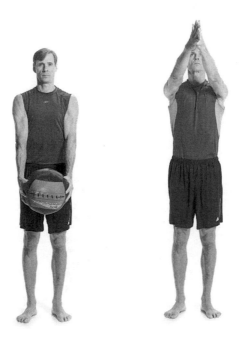

Stand straight upright in a parallel stance with your feet spaced shoulder-width apart. Hold the ball out in front of your body at abdomen level with a firm grip and with your arms extended. Forcefully lift your arms straight up, keeping your elbows straight, then release the ball, double-clap your hands, and catch the ball. Lower the ball with control, and rhythmically repeat the tosses and catches.

Straight-Arm Toss, Side Twist, Jump, and Catch

Benefits: Improves quickness and footwork; strengthens ankles, feet, knees, and hips; strengthens abdominal muscles; improves hand-eye coordination and timing.

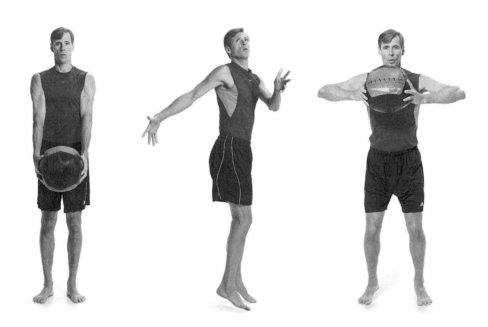

Stand with your feet in a parallel stance, spaced shoulder-width apart. Hold the ball with a firm grip, with your arms extended in front of your abdomen. Throw the ball straight up, then quickly jump and turn to the left. While the ball is still in the air, jump back to your original position and catch the ball before it drops past your chest. Repeat to the other direction. Doing this in each direction equals one repetition.

Single-Leg Ball Passing

Benefits: Improves balance and hand-eye coordination; strengthens hip flexors and forearms; and improves hamstring flexibility.

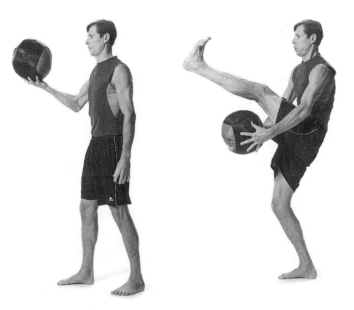

Stand upright in a split stance with your right leg forward. Hold the ball in your right hand in front of you. Swing your left leg toward the ceiling while keeping it fully extended. Quickly pass the ball under your left leg to your left hand. Lower your leg to the floor, then switch the ball back to your right hand. Complete all repetitions with the left leg, then change your stance and repeat on the other side.

Single Leg and Arm Extensions

Benefits: Improves your balance and coordination; strengthens abdominal, back, triceps, and shoulder muscles; and provides strength and endurance in the muscles of your feet, knees, hips, and thighs.

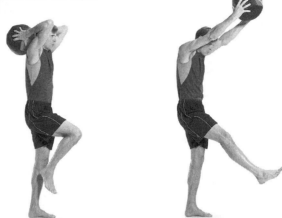

Stand on your left leg, with your right knee bent and lifted in front of you. Firmly hold the ball behind your head. Straighten your arms up toward the ceiling, while simultaneously extending your right leg out in front of you. Energetically exhale while extending. Inhale deeply, exhale, and lower the ball and your leg. Complete all repetitions with one leg. Recover a moment, and repeat with the other leg.

Norman Adler

After only 4 months of doing sessions of *Four Way Burn* techniques twice a week, Norman Adler had already noticed major improvements in his performance on the tennis court.

"I've been playing for years and years. Now, I stand in a more balanced position and I can get to the ball better. And my reflexes are much better. When I hit the shot, I have more 'oomph,'" he says.

The 74-year-old has noticed improvements that make his life better off the court, too. "My posture was declining, and now it's better. My muscles are suppler, and I just feel better."

Norman quickly discovered that focusing his mind on the weighted ball as he moves it around his body offers benefits that he won't get from any other conditioning program.

"While you're holding the Performance Ball, you have to be on balance—you can't stray. You work with your mind and your body, and if you lose your concentration, the exercise goes off the mark. If your mind is wandering, Ralf picks up on it and asks if you can feel what you're doing wrong," he says.

His improved focus—as well as his balance, reflexes, and strong muscles—will help ensure that he sends the ball back over the net with plenty of "oomph" for years to come.

TENNIS CONDITIONING CHART

CYCLE ONE (2 WEEKS)	CYCLE TWO (2 WEEKS)	CYCLE THREE (2 WEEKS)
Pull and Chop 15 reps toward each side	Knead and Jump 3 times (15 seconds) each leg	Quick Feet Push and Pull 15 seconds of foot-shuffling
Rocking Chair 15 reps	Triple Jump, Back Lunge, and Side Twist 10 times on each side	Straight-Arm Toss, Hand Clap, and Catch 20 reps
Repeat the first two exercises for a second set, then move to the next three.		
Race Car Driver 10 reps in each direction	Squat and Racket Reach 10 times in each direction	Straight-Arm Toss, Side Twist, Jump, and Catch 5 reps
Triple Jump, Forward Lunge, and Side Twist 10 reps on each side	Jump and Twist 20 reps in each direction	Single-Leg Ball Passing 10 reps on each side
Alternating Diagonal Lunge and Reach 10 reps on each side	Side Shuffle, Drop, Clap, and Catch 5 shuffles from side to side, each side	Single Leg and Arm Extensions 15 reps with each leg
Repeat the second three exercises for a second set, then move to the relaxation/stretching techniques below. (See pages 41 to 43.)		
Wedge	Wedge	Wedge
Lying Side Twist	Lying Side Twist	Lying Side Twist
Spread Eagle	Spread Eagle	Spread Eagle

Appendix

The strength and flexibility gains you get from the *Four Way Burn* program will improve your ability to do any physical activity that you encounter during the day. However, you should notice particular improvements in certain movements and activities from certain techniques.

The following lists will highlight the particular benefits you'll get from these techniques in your daily life and your sporting activities.

Archery: Dough Kneading, Hula Hoop, Knee Tuck and Push, Push and Pull, Side Twist

Baseball and softball (including other throwing and catching activities): Advanced Push and Pull, Atlas, Around the World, Back Lunge with Double Twist and Kick, Behind-the-Leg Pass, Carioca Loop, The Coil, Crescent Reach, Diagonal Chop, Discus, Dough Kneading, Figure Eight Walk, Front-Arm Raise with Leg Abduction, Good Morning, Good Morning with Side Twist, Hula Hoop, Knee Tuck and Push, Triceps and Leg Extensions, Leg Extensions, Opposite Reach, Mower, Overhead Juggling, Pecking Bird, Power Jacks, Push and Pull, Race Car Driver, Rocking Chair, Saturn, Side Twist, Soldier Walk, Spider Walk, Split Stand Reach to Toes, Squat and Push, Statue of Liberty, Thigh Kick and Catch, Twist and Sweep, Way Down and Way Up

Basketball: Around the World, Atlas, Back Lunge with Double Twist and Kick, Behind-the-Leg Pass, Carioca Loop, Crescent Reach, Diagonal Chop, Discus, Dough Kneading, Figure Eight Walk, Front-Arm Raise with Leg Abduction, Golfer Swing, Good Morning, Good Morning with Side Twist, Knee Lift and Side Twist, Knee Tuck and Push, Leg Extension Opposite Reach, Mower, Overhead Juggling, Pecking Bird, Power Jacks, Race Car Driver, Rocking Chair, Saturn, Side Twist, Spider Walk, Split Stand Reach to Toes, Squat and Push, Statue of Liberty, Straddle Squat and Reach, Thigh Kick and Catch, Thigh Kick and Soldier Walk, Triceps and Leg Extensions, Twist and Sweep, Way Down and Way Up

Bending or squatting: Atlas, Behind-the-Leg Pass, The Coil, Front-Arm Raise with Leg Abduction, Pecking Bird, Split Stand Reach to Toes, Squat and Push, Straddle Squat and Reach, Way Down and Way Up

Bicycling: See Chapter 11.

Billiards: Dough Kneading, Good Morning, Push and Pull, Race Car Driver

Bowling: Advanced Push and Pull, Atlas, Back Lunge with Double Twist and Kick, Behind-the-Leg Pass, Carioca Loop, The Coil, Discus, Dough Kneading, Figure Eight Walk, Front-Arm Raise with Leg Abduction, Good Morning, Good Morning with Side Twist, Hula Hoop, Knee Lift and Side Twist, Knee Tuck and Push, Leg Extension Opposite Reach, Mower, Pecking Bird, Power Jacks, Push and Pull, Race Car Driver, Side Twist, Soldier Walk, Spider Walk, Split Stand Reach to Toes, Squat and Push, Straddle Squat and Reach, Thigh Kick and Soldier Walk, Triceps and Leg Extensions, Twist and Sweep

Boxing: Back Lunge with Double Twist and Kick, Crescent Reach, Discus, Dough Kneading, Front-Arm Raise with Leg Abduction, Golfer Swing, Hula Hoop, Overhead Juggling, Pecking Bird, Power Jacks, Push and Pull, Saturn, Side Twist

Canoeing and kayaking: Crescent Reach, Knee Tuck and Push

Caring for animals: Advanced Push and Pull, Around the World, Atlas, Back Lunge with Double Twist and Kick, Behind-the-Leg Pass, The Coil, Crescent Reach, Discus, Figure Eight Walk, Front-Arm Raise with Leg Abduction, Good Morning with Side Twist, Knee Tuck and Push, Power Jacks, Push and Pull, Race Car Driver, Side Twist, Split Stand Reach to Toes, Squat and Push, Straddle Squat and Reach, Triceps and Leg Extensions, Way Down and Way Up

Carrying loads: Advanced Push and Pull, Crescent Reach, Knee Lift and Side Twist, Leg Extension Opposite Reach, Pecking Bird, Soldier Walk, Spider Walk, Statue of Liberty, Straddle Squat and Reach, Thigh Kick and Soldier Walk

Child care: Atlas, Back Lunge with Double Twist and Kick, Behind-the-Leg Pass, Carioca Loop, The Coil, Crescent Reach, Figure Eight Walk, Front-Arm Raise with Leg Abduction, Good Morning, Good Morning with Side Twist, Knee Lift and Side Twist, Knee Tuck and Push, Mower, Pecking Bird, Power Jacks, Push and Pull, Spider Walk, Split Stand Reach to Toes, Squat and Push, Straddle Squat and Reach, Triceps and Leg Extensions, Way Down and Way Up

Climbing ladders and stairs: Advanced Push and Pull, Back Lunge with Double Twist and Kick, Knee Lift and Side Twist, Leg Extension Opposite Reach, Thigh Kick and Catch, Thigh Kick and Soldier Walk

Curling: Behind-the-Leg Pass, Dough Kneading, Twist and Sweep

Dancing: Carioca Loop, Front-Arm Raise with Leg Abduction, Mower, Side Twist

Diving: Crescent Reach, Discus, Good Morning, Hula Hoop, Mower, Push and Pull, Race Car Driver, Rocking Chair, Saturn, Soldier Walk, Triceps and Leg Extensions, Way Down and Way Up

Dressing: Back Lunge with Double Twist and Kick, Behind-the-Leg Pass, Carioca Loop, The Coil, Crescent Reach, Diagonal Chop, Front-Arm Raise with Leg Abduction, Good Morning, Good

Morning with Side Twist, Hula Hoop, Knee Lift and Side Twist, Knee Tuck and Push, Leg Extension Opposite Reach, Pecking Bird, Push and Pull, Race Car Driver, Saturn, Split Stand Reach to Toes, Statue of Liberty, Straddle Squat and Reach, Triceps and Leg Extensions

Driving and getting in and out of a car: Diagonal Chop, Dough Kneading, Front-Arm Raise with Leg Abduction, Good Morning with Side Twist, Hula Hoop, Knee Lift and Side Twist, Knee Tuck and Push, Pecking Bird, Push and Pull, Race Car Driver, Side Twist, Squat and Push

Equestrian sports: Around the World, Dough Kneading, Hula Hoop, Push and Pull, Race Car Driver, Side Twist, Split Stand Reach to Toes, Squat and Push, Straddle Squat and Reach, Twist and Sweep

Fencing: Advanced Push and Pull, Back Lunge with Double Twist and Kick, Behind-the-Leg Pass, Dough Kneading, Hula Hoop, Knee Tuck and Push, Pecking Bird, Power Jacks, Race Car Driver, Thigh Kick and Soldier Walk, Twist and Sweep

Fishing: Advanced Push and Pull, Around the World, Crescent Reach, Discus, Dough Kneading, Front-Arm Raise with Leg Abduction, Knee Tuck and Push, Race Car Driver, Saturn, Side Twist, Straddle Squat and Reach, Triceps and Leg Extensions

Football: Advanced Push and Pull, Around the World, Atlas, Back Lunge with Double Twist and Kick, Behind-the-Leg Pass, Carioca Loop, The Coil, Crescent Reach, Dough Kneading, Figure Eight Walk, Front-Arm Raise with Leg Abduction, Good Morning with Side Twist, Knee Tuck and Push, Knee Lift and Side Twist, Leg Extension Opposite Reach, Overhead Juggling, Pecking Bird, Power Jacks, Push and Pull, Race Car Driver, Rocking Chair, Saturn, Side Twist, Spider Walk, Statue of Liberty, Straddle Squat and Reach, Thigh Kick and Catch, Thigh Kick and Soldier Walk, Triceps and Leg Extensions, Way Down and Way Up

Gardening (including raking): Advanced Push and Pull, Atlas, Back Lunge with Double Twist and Kick, Behind-the-Leg Pass, Carioca Loop, The Coil, Discus, Dough Kneading, Figure Eight Walk, Golfer Swing, Good Morning, Hula Hoop, Knee Lift and Side Twist, Knee Tuck and Push, Leg Extension Opposite Reach, Push and Pull, Side Twist, Soldier Walk, Spider Walk, Split Stand Reach to Toes, Squat and Push, Straddle Squat and Reach, Way Down and Way Up

Golf: See Chapter 12.

Gymnastics: Advanced Push and Pull, Around the World, Atlas, Back Lunge with Double Twist and Kick, Carioca Loop, The Coil, Diagonal Chop, Discus, Dough Kneading, Figure Eight Walk, Front-Arm Raise with Leg Abduction, Golfer Swing, Good Morning, Good Morning with Side Twist, Hula Hoop, Knee Tuck and Push, Leg Extension Opposite Reach, Mower, Pecking Bird, Power Jacks, Race Car Driver, Rocking Chair, Side Twist, Soldier Walk, Split Stand Reach to Toes, Straddle Squat and Reach, Thigh Kick and Catch, Thigh Kick and Soldier Walk, Triceps and Leg Extensions, Twist and Sweep, Way Down and Way Up

Handball: Advanced Push and Pull, Back Lunge with Double Twist and Kick, Carioca Loop, Diagonal Chop, Discus, Front-Arm Raise with Leg Abduction, Hula Hoop, Knee Tuck and Push, Pecking Bird, Push and Pull, Race Car Driver, Rocking Chair, Split Stand Reach to Toes, Statue of Liberty, Thigh Kick and Catch, Thigh Kick and Soldier Walk, Way Down and Way Up

Hiking: Atlas, Behind-the-Leg Pass, Front-Arm Raise with Leg Abduction, Rocking Chair, Soldier Walk, Thigh Kick and Soldier Walk

Hockey: Advanced Push and Pull, Around the World, Atlas, Back Lunge with Double Twist and Kick, Behind-the-Leg Pass, Carioca Loop, The Coil, Diagonal Chop, Discus, Dough Kneading, Figure Eight Walk, Front-Arm Raise with Leg Abduction, Golfer Swing, Good Morning, Good Morning with Side Twist, Knee Lift and Side Twist, Knee Tuck and Push, Leg Extension Opposite Reach, Overhead Juggling, Pecking Bird, Power Jacks, Push and Pull, Race Car Driver, Rocking Chair, Side Twist, Soldier Walk, Spider Walk, Split Stand Reach to Toes, Squat and Push, Statue of Liberty, Straddle Squat and Reach, Thigh Kick and Catch, Thigh Kick and Soldier Walk, Twist and Sweep, Way Down and Way Up

Home chores (including cooking, changing bedsheets, mopping, sweeping, vacuuming, snow shoveling, painting, washing the car): Atlas, Advanced Push and Pull, Back Lunge with Double Twist and Kick, Behind-the-Leg Pass, Carioca Loop, The Coil, Diagonal Chop, Discus, Dough Kneading, Figure Eight Walk, Front-Arm Raise with Leg Abduction, Golfer Swing, Good Morning, Good Morning with Side Twist, Hula Hoop, Knee Lift and Side Twist, Knee Tuck and Push, Pecking Bird, Power Jacks, Push and Pull, Race Car Driver, Saturn, Side Twist, Soldier Walk, Spider Walk, Squat and Push, Straddle Squat and Reach, Triceps and Leg Extensions, Twist and Sweep

Jumping: Pecking Bird, Rocking Chair, Way Down and Way Up

Lacrosse: Advanced Push and Pull, Around the World, Atlas, Back Lunge with Double Twist and Kick, Behind-the-Leg Pass, Carioca Loop, The Coil, Diagonal Chop, Discus, Figure Eight Walk, Front-Arm Raise with Leg Abduction, Golfer Swing, Good Morning, Good Morning with Side Twist, Knee Lift and Side Twist, Knee Tuck and Push, Leg Extension Opposite Reach, Overhead Juggling, Pecking Bird, Race Car Driver, Soldier Walk, Spider Walk, Split Stand Reach to Toes, Squat and Push, Statue of Liberty, Twist and Sweep, Way Down and Way Up

Lifting: Around the World, Back Lunge with Double Twist and Kick, The Coil, Diagonal Chop, Discus, Good Morning, Hula Hoop, Push and Pull, Split Stand Reach to Toes

Lifting, power lifting: Rocking Chair, Soldier Walk, Spider Walk, Straddle Squat and Reach

Lifting, weight lifting: Dough Kneading, Good Morning, Hula Hoop, Power Jacks, Push and Pull, Rocking Chair, Saturn, Squat and Push

Martial arts, including kickboxing: Advanced Push and Pull, Around the World, Back Lunge with Double Twist and Kick, Behind-the-Leg Pass, Carioca Loop, The Coil, Crescent Reach, Diagonal

Chop, Dough Kneading, Figure Eight Walk, Golfer Swing, Good Morning, Good Morning with Side Twist, Hula Hoop, Knee Lift and Side Twist, Knee Tuck and Push, Leg Extension Opposite Reach, Overhead Juggling, Pecking Bird, Push and Pull, Race Car Driver, Rocking Chair, Saturn, Side Twist, Soldier Walk, Spider Walk, Split Stand Reach to Toes, Squat and Push, Statue of Liberty, Straddle Squat and Reach, Thigh Kick and Catch, Thigh Kick and Soldier Walk, Triceps and Leg Extensions, Twist and Sweep, Way Down and Way Up

Parachuting: Crescent Reach, Dough Kneading, Triceps and Leg Extensions

Pulling: Discus, Dough Kneading, Hula Hoop, Leg Extension Opposite Reach, Push and Pull, Race Car Driver, Split Stand Reach to Toes, Squat and Push

Pushing: Push and Pull, Squat and Push, Hula Hoop, Dough Kneading, Thigh Kick and Soldier Walk, Race Car Driver

Racket sports, badminton: Back Lunge with Double Twist and Kick, Carioca Loop, Crescent Reach, Diagonal Chop, Dough Kneading, Figure Eight Walk, Front-Arm Raise with Leg Abduction, Good Morning, Good Morning with Side Twist, Hula Hoop, Knee Lift and Side Twist, Knee Tuck and Push, Leg Extension Opposite Reach, Mower, Pecking Bird, Power Jacks, Push and Pull, Race Car Driver, Rocking Chair, Saturn, Side Twist, Spider Walk, Split Stand Reach to Toes, Statue of Liberty, Triceps and Leg Extensions, Way Down and Way Up

Racket sports, racquetball: Advanced Push and Pull, Atlas, Back Lunge with Double Twist and Kick, Carioca Loop, The Coil, Crescent Reach, Diagonal Chop, Discus, Dough Kneading, Figure Eight Walk, Front-Arm Raise with Leg Abduction, Golfer Swing, Good Morning, Good Morning with Side Twist, Hula Hoop, Knee Lift and Side Twist, Leg Extension Opposite Reach, Mower, Overhead Juggling, Pecking Bird, Power Jacks, Push and Pull, Race Car Driver, Rocking Chair, Side Twist, Soldier Walk, Spider Walk, Split Stand Reach to Toes, Statue of Liberty, Straddle Squat and Reach, Thigh Kick and Catch, Thigh Kick and Soldier Walk, Triceps and Leg Extensions, Twist and Sweep, Way Down and Way Up

Racket sports, squash: Advanced Push and Pull, Around the World, Atlas, Back Lunge with Double Twist and Kick, Behind-the-Leg Pass, Carioca Loop, The Coil, Crescent Reach, Diagonal Chop, Discus, Dough Kneading, Figure Eight Walk, Front-Arm Raise with Leg Abduction, Golfer Swing, Good Morning, Good Morning with Side Twist, Hula Hoop, Knee Lift and Side Twist, Knee Tuck and Push, Leg Extension Opposite Reach, Mower, Overhead Juggling, Pecking Bird, Power Jacks, Push and Pull, Race Car Driver, Rocking Chair, Side Twist, Soldier Walk, Spider Walk, Split Stand Reach to Toes, Squat and Push, Statue of Liberty, Thigh Kick and Catch, Thigh Kick and Soldier Walk, Triceps and Leg Extensions, Way Down and Way Up

Racket sports, table tennis: Advanced Push and Pull, Figure Eight Walk, Front-Arm Raise with Leg Abduction, Golfer Swing, Good Morning, Good Morning with Side Twist, Side Twist

Racket sports, tennis: See Chapter 13.

Reaching: Advanced Push and Pull, Atlas, Back Lunge with Double Twist and Kick, Behind-the-Leg Pass, Crescent Reach, Diagonal Chop, Discus, Leg Extension Opposite Reach, Mower, Pecking Bird, Race Car Driver, Rocking Chair, Split Stand Reach to Toes, Straddle Squat and Reach

Reaching, overhead: Figure Eight Walk, Good Morning, Hula Hoop, Mower, Overhead Juggling, Push and Pull, Triceps and Leg Extensions

Recreational vehicle driving (including motorcycles, jet skis, snowmobiles): Advanced Push and Pull, Around the World, Crescent Reach, Discus, Dough Kneading, Golfer Swing, Good Morning, Good Morning with Side Twist, Knee Tuck and Push, Power Jacks, Push and Pull, Saturn, Side Twist, Soldier Walk, Split Stand Reach to Toes, Squat and Push, Straddle Squat and Reach, Rocking Chair

Rock climbing: Around the World, Back Lunge with Double Twist and Kick, Crescent Reach, Diagonal Chop, Dough Kneading, Figure Eight Walk, Front-Arm Raise with Leg Abduction, Hula Hoop, Knee Lift and Side Twist, Knee Tuck and Push, Leg Extension Opposite Reach, Mower, Overhead Juggling, Pecking Bird, Race Car Driver, Rocking Chair, Soldier Walk, Spider Walk, Statue of Liberty, Thigh Kick and Soldier Walk, Twist and Sweep, Way Down and Way Up

Rowing: Advanced Push and Pull, Atlas, Crescent Reach, Good Morning, Good Morning with Side Twist, Hula Hoop, Pecking Bird, Push and Pull, Split Stand Reach to Toes, Squat and Push, Straddle Squat and Reach

Rugby: Atlas, Back Lunge with Double Twist and Kick, Carioca Loop, Diagonal Chop, Discus, Figure Eight Walk, Front-Arm Raise with Leg Abduction, Knee Tuck and Push, Leg Extension Opposite Reach, Mower, Overhead Juggling, Squat and Push, Way Down and Way Up

Running/Jogging: Advanced Push and Pull, Behind-the-Leg Pass, Carioca Loop, Rocking Chair, Side Twist, Soldier Walk, Spider Walk, Split Stand Reach to Toes, Statue of Liberty, Thigh Kick and Catch, Thigh Kick and Soldier Walk. See also Chapter 10.

Sailing: Front-Arm Raise with Leg Abduction, Good Morning with Side Twist, Leg Extension Opposite Reach, Overhead Juggling, Race Car Driver, Side Twist, Split Stand Reach to Toes, Triceps and Leg Extensions

Sex: Front-Arm Raise with Leg Abduction, Good Morning, Hula Hoop, Push and Pull, Spider Walk, Squat and Push, Triceps and Leg Extensions, Way Down and Way Up

Shopping: Advanced Push and Pull, Behind-the-Leg Pass, The Coil, Crescent Reach, Discus, Dough Kneading, Good Morning, Hula Hoop, Leg Extension Opposite Reach, Pecking Bird, Push and Pull, Race Car Driver, Saturn, Squat and Push, Thigh Kick and Catch

Showering and bathing: Atlas, Back Lunge with Double Twist and Kick, Behind-the-Leg Pass, The Coil, Crescent Reach, Discus, Diagonal Chop, Dough Kneading, Figure Eight Walk, Front-Arm

Raise with Leg Abduction, Good Morning, Good Morning with Side Twist, Hula Hoop, Knee Lift and Side Twist, Knee Tuck and Push, Leg Extension Opposite Reach, Pecking Bird, Push and Pull, Race Car Driver, Rocking Chair, Saturn, Spider Walk, Squat and Push, Statue of Liberty, Straddle Squat and Reach, Thigh Kick and Catch, Thigh Kick and Soldier Walk, Triceps and Leg Extensions

Sitting and standing activities, including desk and computer work: Around the World, The Coil, Hula Hoop, Saturn, Squat and Push, Twist and Sweep

Skateboarding: Atlas, Diagonal Chop, Discus, Figure Eight Walk, Front-Arm Raise with Leg Abduction, Golfer Swing, Pecking Bird, Power Jacks, Push and Pull, Race Car Driver, Side Twist, Spider Walk, Split Stand Reach to Toes, Twist and Sweep

Skating, including figure skating and roller skating: Back Lunge with Double Twist and Kick, Behind-the-Leg Pass, Carioca Loop, Crescent Reach, Diagonal Chop, Dough Kneading, Front-Arm Raise with Leg Abduction, Golfer Swing, Good Morning, Knee Lift and Side Twist, Knee Tuck and Push, Leg Extension Opposite Reach, Mower, Race Car Driver, Rocking Chair, Saturn, Side Twist, Soldier Walk, Squat and Push, Statue of Liberty, Straddle Squat and Reach, Twist and Sweep, Way Down and Way Up

Skiing: Around the World, Behind-the-Leg Pass, Carioca Loop, The Coil, Discus, Dough Kneading, Figure Eight Walk, Good Morning, Good Morning with Side Twist, Hula Hoop, Knee Lift and Side Twist, Knee Tuck and Push, Leg Extension Opposite Reach, Mower, Pecking Bird, Power Jacks, Rocking Chair, Spider Walk, Split Stand Reach to Toes, Statue of Liberty, Triceps and Leg Extensions, Twist and Sweep, Way Down and Way Up

Skiing, alpine: Push and Pull, Saturn, Side Twist, Squat and Push

Skiing, cross-country: Advanced Push and Pull, Back Lunge with Double Twist and Kick, Behind-the-Leg Pass, Dough Kneading, Hula Hoop, Leg Extension Opposite Reach, Mower, Pecking Bird, Push and Pull, Race Car Driver, Rocking Chair, Side Twist, Soldier Walk, Thigh Kick and Soldier Walk, Triceps and Leg Extensions, Twist and Sweep

Skiing, freestyle: Soldier Walk, Twist and Sweep

Skiing, ski jumping: Rocking Chair, Spider Walk

Skiing, water: Advanced Push and Pull, Around the World, Back Lunge with Double Twist and Kick, Behind-the-Leg Pass, Crescent Reach, Discus, Dough Kneading, Front-Arm Raise with Leg Abduction, Good Morning, Good Morning with Side Twist, Hula Hoop, Leg Extension Opposite Reach, Pecking Bird, Power Jacks, Push and Pull, Race Car Driver, Side Twist, Soldier Walk, Spider Walk, Split Stand Reach to Toes, Squat and Push, Straddle Squat and Reach, Triceps and Leg Extensions, Way Down and Way Up

Sledding, including bobsledding: Advanced Push and Pull, Around the World, Behind-the-Leg Pass, Power Jacks, Spider Walk, Squat and Push

Snowboarding: Atlas, Diagonal Chop, Discus, Dough Kneading, Figure Eight Walk, Front-Arm Raise with Leg Abduction, Golfer Swing, Good Morning, Good Morning with Side Twist, Power Jacks, Push and Pull, Side Twist, Spider Walk, Split Stand Reach to Toes, Squat and Push, Straddle Squat and Reach, Race Car Driver, Rocking Chair, Twist and Sweep

Soccer: Advanced Push and Pull, Around the World, Atlas, Back Lunge with Double Twist and Kick, Behind-the-Leg Pass, Carioca Loop, Crescent Reach, Diagonal Chop, Discus, Dough Kneading, Figure Eight Walk, Front-Arm Raise with Leg Abduction, Golfer Swing, Good Morning with Side Twist, Hula Hoop, Knee Lift and Side Twist, Knee Tuck and Push, Leg Extension Opposite Reach, Mower, Overhead Juggling, Pecking Bird, Power Jacks, Push and Pull, Race Car Driver, Rocking Chair, Saturn, Side Twist, Soldier Walk, Spider Walk, Split Stand Reach to Toes, Statue of Liberty, Straddle Squat and Reach, Thigh Kick and Catch, Twist and Sweep, Way Down and Way Up

Surfing: Back Lunge with Double Twist and Kick, The Coil, Crescent Reach, Diagonal Chop, Discus, Figure Eight Walk, Golfer Swing, Good Morning, Good Morning with Side Twist, Overhead Juggling, Pecking Bird, Race Car Driver, Side Twist, Spider Walk, Split Stand Reach to Toes, Squat and Push, Straddle Squat and Reach, Triceps and Leg Extensions, Way Down and Way Up

Swimming: Around the World, Atlas, The Coil, Crescent Reach, Dough Kneading, Golfer Swing, Hula Hoop, Mower, Overhead Juggling, Race Car Driver, Rocking Chair, Saturn, Side Twist, Triceps and Leg Extensions, Twist and Sweep

Track and field: Around the World, Atlas, Back Lunge with Double Twist and Kick, Carioca Loop, The Coil, Crescent Reach, Diagonal Chop, Discus, Dough Kneading, Figure Eight Walk, Front-Arm Raise with Leg Abduction, Good Morning, Good Morning with Side Twist, Knee Lift and Side Twist, Knee Tuck and Push, Leg Extension Opposite Reach, Mower, Pecking Bird, Push and Pull, Race Car Driver, Saturn, Side Twist, Soldier Walk, Spider Walk, Split Stand Reach to Toes, Squat and Push, Statue of Liberty, Straddle Squat and Reach, Thigh Kick and Soldier Walk, Triceps and Leg Extensions, Way Down and Way Up

Track and field, hurdles: Behind-the-Leg Pass

Track and field, long jump: Behind-the-Leg Pass

Trampoline: The Coil, Golfer Swing, Good Morning with Side Twist, Power Jacks, Race Car Driver, Rocking Chair

Traveling: Hula Hoop, Push and Pull, Saturn, Side Twist

Volleyball: Advanced Push and Pull, Around the World, Back Lunge with Double Twist and Kick, Carioca Loop, The Coil, Crescent Reach, Diagonal Chop, Discus, Dough Kneading, Figure Eight

Walk, Front-Arm Raise with Leg Abduction, Good Morning with Side Twist, Hula Hoop, Knee Lift and Side Twist, Knee Tuck and Push, Leg Extension Opposite Reach, Mower, Overhead Juggling, Pecking Bird, Power Jacks, Race Car Driver, Rocking Chair, Saturn, Side Twist, Soldier Walk, Spider Walk, Split Stand Reach to Toes, Squat and Push, Statue of Liberty, Straddle Squat and Reach, Thigh Kick and Catch, Triceps and Leg Extensions, Way Down and Way Up

Walking, including hiking: Advanced Push and Pull, Behind-the-Leg Pass, Carioca Loop, Knee Lift and Side Twist, Rocking Chair, Side Twist, Soldier Walk, Spider Walk, Split Stand Reach to Toes, Statue of Liberty, Thigh Kick and Catch, Thigh Kick and Soldier Walk. See also Chapter 10.

Walking over uneven surfaces: Around the World, Back Lunge with Double Twist and Kick, Pecking Bird, Statue of Liberty

Water polo: Leg Extension Opposite Reach, Mower, Side Twist

Windsurfing: Advanced Push and Pull, Behind-the-Leg Pass, Crescent Reach, Dough Kneading, Figure Eight Walk, Front-Arm Raise with Leg Abduction, Good Morning, Good Morning with Side Twist, Leg Extension Opposite Reach, Overhead Juggling, Pecking Bird, Push and Pull, Race Car Driver, Side Twist, Split Stand Reach to Toes, Straddle Squat and Reach, Triceps and Leg Extensions

Wrestling: Crescent Reach, Figure Eight Walk, Front-Arm Raise with Leg Abduction, Knee Tuck and Push, Leg Extension Opposite Reach, Overhead Juggling, Pecking Bird, Race Car Driver, Split Stand Reach to Toes, Straddle Squat and Reach

Index

Boldface page references indicate photographs. <u>Underscored</u> references indicate boxed text and charts.

A

Abdominal muscles
   in cycling, 175
   strengthening, for reducing back problems, 119
   in tennis, 227
Adler, Norman, <u>244</u>
Aerobic exercise, 19, 121. *See also specific sport*
Alpine skiing, 253
Animal care activities, 248
Ankles
   in cycling, 176
   in tennis, 228
Archery, 247
Arms
   Four Way Burn program benefits and, 20
   in tennis, 227

B

Back. *See also* Back problems
   stretching, 90–92
   in tennis, 227

Back problems
   causes of
      sedentary lifestyle, 117
      stress, 118
      weight, 5, 118
   Four Way Burn program techniques and benefits of, 8, 121
   Bridging, 129, **129**
   chart, <u>142–44</u>
   cycles of, completing, 121
   Good Morning with Side Twist, 137, **137**
   Knee Tuck and Push, 139, **139**
   Lying Side Twist, 126, **126**
   Reach, Tuck, and Touch, 125, **125**
   Seated Good Morning, 123, **123**
   Seated Pass to Yourself, 141, **141**
   Seated Side Twist, 122, **122**
   Side Twist, 127, **127**
   Single-Leg Raise and Crunch, 140, **140**
   Situp, Knee Lift, and Twist, 135, **135**
   Sit Up and Pass the Ball, 136, **136**
   Sit Up and Reach, 131, **131**
   Squat and Hold, 134, **134**
   Squat and Push, 138, **138**
   Squat and Reach, 128, **128**
   Straddle Squat and Reach, 133, **133**

Back problems (*cont.*)
   Four Way Burn program
      techniques and (*cont.*)
        Three Way Hip, 130, **130**
        Twist and Sweep, 132, **132**
        Wall Squat, 124, **124**
   physical activity and, 120–21
   reducing with
      body alignment, 119–20
      ergonomics, 120
      flexibility, 119
      good posture, 119–20
      strong muscles, 119
   rest and, myth of, 120
Badminton, 251
Balance, dynamic, 199
Baseball, 247
Basketball, 247
Bathing activities, 252–53
Beach ball, 21–22
Bending activities, 247
Bikes, 10, 197. *See also* Cycling
Billiards, 248
Bobsledding, 254
Body alignment, 119–20
Body fat percentage, 115
Bowling, 248
Boxing, 248
Browne, Carol, 14
Buffer zone, 8
Buttocks muscles
   in cycling, 175
   in walking and running, 148

C

Calorie burning, 19, 113
Calorie consumption, 106
Calves, in cycling, 176
Cancer, 4
Canoeing, 248

Cardiovascular fitness, 13, 18
Car driving, 249
Carrying activities, 248
Catching activities, 247
Charts for *Four Way Burn*
      program techniques
   back problems, 142–44
   Cycle 1, 44
   Cycle 2, 57
   Cycle 3, 69
   Cycle 4, 84
   cycling, 198
   golf, 225
   tennis, 245
   traveling, 104
   walking and running, 173
Child care activities, 248
Climbing activities, 248
Conditioning, mental and physical, 18
Cooldowns, 23
Core muscles
   Four Way Burn program
      benefits and, 20
   in golf, 199
   "multitasking" and, 12
Cross-country skiing, 253
Curling, 248
Cycle 1 of *Four Way Burn* program
   personal experience, 30
   starting levels, 28–29
   techniques
      chart, 44
      Discus, 40, **40**
      Good Morning, 39, **39**
      Hula Hoop, 36, **36**
      Lying Side Twist, 42, **42**
      Push and Pull, 31, **31**
      Rocking Chair, 34, **34**
      Saturn, 32, **32**
      Side Twist, 33, **33**
      Soldier Walk, 38, **38**
      Spread Eagle, 43, **43**
      Squat and Push, 35, **35**

Thigh Kick and Catch, 37, **37**
Wedge, 41, **41**
tips, 27, 30
Cycle 2 of *Four Way Burn* program
overview, 45
techniques
Advanced Push and Pull, 48,
48
Behind-the-Leg Pass, 55, **55**
chart, <u>57</u>
Coil, 46–47, **46–47**
Diagonal Chop, 49, **49**
Dough Kneading, 53, **53**
Golfer Swing, 50, **50**
Power Jacks, 52, **52**
Spider Walk, 54, **54**
Statue of Liberty, 51, **51**
Twist and Sweep, 56, **56**
Cycle 3 of *Four Way Burn* program
overview, 58
techniques
Around the World, 65, **65**
Atlas, 62, **62**
Carioca Loop, 60, **60**
chart, <u>69</u>
Knee Lift and Side Twist, 59, **59**
Leg Extension Opposite Reach, 66, **66**
Mower, 67, **67**
Overhead Juggling, 64, **64**
Split Stand Reach to Toes, 68, **68**
Straddle Squat and Reach, 61, **61**
Thigh Kick and Soldier Walk, 63, **63**
Cycle 4 of *Four Way Burn* program
completion of, 82
overview, 70
techniques
Back Lunge with Double Twist and Kick,
78, **78**
chart, <u>84</u>
Crescent Reach, 76, **76**
Figure Eight Walk, 74, **74**
Front-Arm Raise with Leg Abduction,
79, **79**

Good Morning with Side Twist, 71, **71**
Knee Tuck and Push, 77, **77**
Pecking Bird, 73, **73**
Race Car Driver, 72, **72**
Triceps and Leg Extensions, 75, **75**
Way Down and Way Up, 80–81, **80–81**
Cycling
abdominal muscles in, 175
ankles in, 176
benefits of, 174
bike fit and, <u>197</u>
buttocks muscles in, 175
calves in, 176
feet in, 176
Four Way Burn program techniques and
Atlas, 191, **191**
benefits of, 8
chart, <u>198</u>
Crescent Reach, 195, **195**
Crunch and Leg Extension, 182, **182**
Dough Kneading, 194, **194**
Good Morning, 183, **183**
Good Morning with Side Twist, 188,
188
Knee Tuck and Push, 196, **196**
Mower, 184, **184**
overview, 176–77
Pecking Bird, 190, **190**
Push and Pull, 178, **178**
Rocking Chair, 189, **189**
Saturn, 179, **179**
sessions, completing, 176–77
Situp, Knee Pull, and Chop, 197, **197**
Situp, Straight-Leg Raise, and Push, 192,
192
Sit Up and Reach Overhead, 187, **187**
Soldier Walk, 185, **185**
Squat and Push, 180, **180**
Straddle Squat and Reach, 186, **186**
Thigh Kick and Catch, 181, **181**
Triceps and Leg Extensions, 193, **193**
hamstrings in, 176
hips in, 175

Cycling (*cont.*)
 injury prevention, 174–76, <u>197</u>
 knees in, 176
 mental component of, 176
 overtraining and, 6–7
 physical challenges of, 175–76
 quadriceps in, 175–76
 senses and, 176
 thighs in, 175–76
 torso in, 175
 upper body in, 175

D

Daily life activities and *Four Way Burn*
  program benefits, 247–55
Dancing, 248
Deep breathing, 18
Depression, 5
Diet and weight loss
 changes, making small,
   107–8
 eating out and, 111–13
 guidelines, 108–10
 low-calorie food, <u>112</u>
 setpoint, finding new, 107
 shopping for food, 111
Distractions, avoiding, 23
Diving, 248
Downhill skiing, 253
Dressing activities, 248–49
Driving activities, 249, 252
Dynamic balance, 199
Dynamic fitness, 6

E

Eating out, 111–13
Emme, <u>17</u>

Endorphins, 21
Equestrian activities, 249
Ergonomics, 120
Exercise, 3, 15, 19, 121. *See also* Physical
  activity; *specific sport*
Extension, 119

F

Feet
 in cycling, 176
 Four Way Burn program in stabilizing, 19
 in mechanics of walking and running, 149
 in tennis, 228
Fencing, 249
Fingers, in tennis, 227
Fishing, 249
Fitness
 buffer zone and, 8
 cardiovascular, 13, 18
 dynamic, 6
 Four Way Burn program benefits and, 7–9,
   18, 21
 fuller, happier life and, 9
 industry, 10–12
 progressive, 15
 pulmonary, 18
 quality of life and, 4–5
 trends, 10
 wellness and, 4
Flexibility
 importance of, 11–12
 physical activity and, 6–7
 reducing back problems and, 119
 sports and, 6
 tennis and, 228
Flexion, 119
Floor technique for posture improvement, 120
Food
 diet guidelines, 108–10
 low-calorie, <u>112</u>

restaurant, 111–13
shopping for, 111
Football, 249
Four Way Burn program. *See also specific cycle*;
    Techniques in *Four Way Burn* program
  advanced level of, 83
  ball used in, 15–16, 21
  barefeet and, 23
  benefits of
    arm movement, 20
    calorie burn, 19
    conditioning, mental and physical, 18
    control of body, 5
    core muscle movement, 20
    in daily activities, 247–55
    feet stabilization, 19
    fitness, 7–9, 18, 21
    joint stability, 8, 18–19
    leg movement, 20
    reducing back problems, 8, 121
    in sporting activities, 6, 8, 247–55
    time needed for, 17
    various other, 20–21
  buffer zone and, 8
  cycles of, 21, 45
  difficulty levels in, 22, 28–29
  distractions and, avoiding, 23
  injury prevention and, 8
  maintenance phase, 82–83
  overview, 7, 16–17
  personal experiences
    Adler, Norman, 244
    Browne, Carol, 14
    Emme, 17
    Handler, Richard, 30
    Madris, Richard, 224
    Simpkins, Nancy, 20
    Weill, Sanford, 9
    Wilkenfeld, Joel, 13
  sessions
    moving through, 22
    taking time with, 24
    timing, 22–23
    starting, 21–24
    stretching incorporated into, 23
    switching sides and, 24
    weight loss and, 116
Freestyle skiing, 253

G

Gardening, 249
Gluteus maximus muscles.
    See Buttocks muscles
Golf
  core muscles in, 199
  dynamic balance and, 199
  Four Way Burn program techniques and
    Around the World, 217, **217**
    Behind-the-Leg Pass, 213, **213**
    benefits of, 8
    Carioca Loop, 215, **215**
    chart, 225
    Coil, 209, **209**
    cycles, completing, 200
    Discus, 208, **208**
    Dough Kneading, 224, **224**
    Figure Eight Walk, 222, **222**
    Front-Arm Raise with Leg Abduction, 223,
      223
    Golfer Swing, 210, **210**
    Good Morning, 207, **207**
    Good Morning with Side Twist, 220, **220**
    Hula Hoop, 204, **204**
    Mower, 218, **218**
    overview, 200
    personal experience, 224
    Push and Pull, 201, **201**
    Race Car Driver, 221, **221**
    Saturn, 202, **202**
    Side Twist, 203, **203**
    Soldier Walk, 206, **206**
    Spider Walk, 212, **212**
    Split Stand Reach to Toes, 219, **219**

Golf (*cont.*)
  Four Way Burn program
      techniques and (*cont.*)
    Squat and Push, 205, **205**
    Statue of Liberty, 211, **211**
    Straddle Squat and Reach, 216, **216**
    Twist and Sweep, 214, **214**
  legs in, 199
  mental aspect of, 200
  overtraining and, 7
  upper body in, 199
Gymnastics, 249

H

Hamstrings
  in cycling, 176
  in mechanics of walking and
      running, 148
Handball, 250
Handler, Richard, <u>30</u>
Hands, in tennis, 227
Heart disease, 4
Heart rate, 18
Hiking, 250, 255. *See also* Walking
      and running
Hips
  in cycling, 175
  in mechanics of walking
      and running, 148
  stretching, 90–92
  in tennis, 228
Hockey, 250
Household chores, 4, 250

I

Ice skating, 253
Injury prevention
  cycling, 174–76, <u>197</u>

Four Way Burn program and, 8
walking and running, 147–48

J

Jogging, 147, 252. *See also* Walking and running
Joint stability, 8, 18–19
Jumping activities, 250

K

Karas, Evan, 6, 19, 120–21
Karate, 16
Kata, 16
Kayaking, 248
Kickboxing, 250–51
Knees
  in cycling, 176
  in mechanics of walking and running, 149

L

Lacrosse, 250
Legs
  Four Way Burn program benefits and, 20
  in golf, 199
  in tennis, 228
Lifting activities, 250
Low-calorie food, <u>112</u>

M

Madris, Richard, <u>224</u>
Maintenance phase, 82–83
Martial arts, 16, 250–51
Medicine ball, 13, 21

Metabolism, 19
Musculoskeletal system and
physical activity, 3–5

N

Neck stretches, 89–90

O

Obesity, 4
Overhead reaching activities,
252
Overtraining, 6–7
Overuse injuries, 6–7
Overweight, 4

P

Parachuting, 251
Performance Ball, 15–16, 21
Physical activity. *See also* Exercise; *specific
activity or sport*
  American attitudes toward, 3
  back problems and, 120–21
  calorie burning and, 113
  flexibility and, 6–7
  lack of, 3–5, 117
  modern conveniences and, 3–4
  musculoskeletal system and,
    3–5
  strength and, 6–7
  traveling and, 87
  varying, 114
  weight loss and, 105, 113–16,
    114
Physical therapy, 10
Pilates, 13

Posture, good, 119–20
Power lifting, 250
Pulling activities, 251
Pulmonary fitness, 18
Pushing activities, 251

Q

Quadriceps
  in cycling, 175–76
  in mechanics of walking and running,
    149
Quality of life, 4–5

R

Racket sports, 251. *See also* Tennis
Racquetball, 251
Raking activities, 249
Range of motion, 19, 119
Reaching activities, 252
Recreational vehicle driving activities,
  252
Recumbent bikes, 10
Resistance methods, 115
Restaurant food, 111–13
Rock climbing, 252
Roller skating, 253
Roller tubes, foam, 10
Rowing, 252
Rugby, 252
Running. *See* Walking and running

S

Sailing, 252
Sex activities, 252
Shopping, 252

Shoulders
    stretching, 89–90
    in tennis, 227
Showering activities, 252–53
Simpkins, Nancy, <u>20</u>
Sitting activities, 253
Skateboarding, 253
Skating, 253
Skiing, 253
Ski jumping, 253
Sledding, 254
Slide boards, 10
Snowboarding, 254
Soccer, 254
Softball, 247
Sporting activities and *Four Way Burn*
    program benefits, 6, 8, 247–55.
    See also specific activity
Squash, 251
Squatting activities, 247
Standing activities, 253
Strength
    joints and, 18–19
    physical activity and, 6–7
    reducing back problems and, 119
    sports and, 6
    tennis and, 228
    weight training and, 11, 115–16, 250
Stress, 5, 118
Stretching
    Four Way Burn program
      techniques and
      incorporation into, 23
      Lying Side Twist, 42, **42**
      Spread Eagle, 43, **43**
      Wedge, 41, **41**
    traveling and
      back, hips, and thighs, 90–92
      neck, shoulders, and upper body,
      89–90
      need for, 88–89
Surfing, 254
Swimming, 254

T

Table tennis, 251
Techniques in *Four Way Burn* program. *See also*
    Charts for *Four Way Burn* program
    techniques
    Advanced Push and Pull, 48, **48**
    Alternating Diagonal Lunge and Reach, 234,
      234
    Around the World
      in Cycle 3, 65, **65**
      golf and, 217, **217**
      traveling and, 102–3, **102–3**
      walking and running and, 155, **155**
    Atlas
      in Cycle 3, 62, **62**
      cycling and, 191, **191**
    Back Lunge Push, Pull, and Side Twist, 158,
      158
    Back Lunge with Double Twist and Kick, 78,
      78
    Behind-the-Leg Pass
      in Cycle 2, 55, **55**
      golf and, 213, **213**
    benefits of, 8, 16
    Bridging, 129, **129**
    Carioca Loop
      in Cycle 3, 60, **60**
      golf and, 215, **215**
      walking and running and, 163, **163**
    Coil
      in Cycle 2, 46–47, **46–47**
      golf and, 209, **209**
      walking and running and, 151–52, **151–52**
    Crescent Reach
      in Cycle 4, 76, **76**
      cycling and, 195, **195**
    Crossover Stand and Reach, 156, **156**
    Crunch and Leg Extension, 182, **182**
    daily life activities' benefits from, 247–55
    Diagonal Chop
      in Cycle 2, 49, **49**
      traveling and, 97, **97**

Discus
in Cycle 1, 40, **40**
golf and, 208, **208**
Dough Kneading
in Cycle 2, 53, **53**
cycling and, 194, **194**
golf and, 224, **224**
Figure Eight Walk
in Cycle 4, 74, **74**
golf and, 222, **222**
Front-Arm Raise with Leg
Abduction
in Cycle 4, 79, **79**
golf and, 223, **223**
traveling and, 96, **96**
walking and running and, 171,
171
Golfer Swing
in Cycle 2, 50, **50**
golf and, 210, **210**
traveling and, 99, **99**
walking and running and, 154,
154
Good Morning
in Cycle 1, 39, **39**
cycling and, 183, **183**
golf and, 207, **207**
Good Morning with Side Twist
back problems and, 137, **137**
in Cycle 4, 71, **71**
cycling and, 188, **188**
golf and, 220, **220**
traveling and, 93, **93**
walking and jogging and, 161, **161**
Hop and Twist, 166, **166**
Hula Hoop
in Cycle 1, 36, **36**
golf and, 204, **204**
Jump and Twist, 238, **238**
Knead and Jump, 235, **235**
Knee Lift and Side Twist
in Cycle 3, 59, **59**
walking and running and, 164, **164**

Knee Tuck and Push
back problems and, 139, **139**
in Cycle 4, 77, **77**
cycling and, 196, **196**
Leg Extension Opposite Reach, 66, **66**
Lying Side Twist
back problems and, 126, **126**
in Cycle 1, 42, **42**
maintenance phase, 82–83
Mower
in Cycle 3, 67, **67**
cycling and, 184, **184**
golf and, 218, **218**
Overhead Juggling, 64, **64**
Pecking Bird
in Cycle 4, 73, **73**
cycling and, 190, **190**
walking and running and, 160, **160**
Power Jacks, 52, **52**
Pull and Chop, 230, **230**
Push and Pull
in Cycle 1, 31, **31**
cycling and, 178, **178**
golf and, 201, **201**
Quick Feet Push and Pull, 240, **240**
Race Car Driver
in Cycle 4, 72, **72**
golf and, 221, **221**
tennis and, 232, **232**
Reach, Tuck, and Touch, 125, **125**
Rocking Chair
in Cycle 1, 34, **34**
cycling and, 189, **189**
tennis and, 231, **231**
traveling and, 101, **101**
walking and running and, 167, **167**
Saturn
in Cycle 1, 32, **32**
cycling and, 179, **179**
golf and, 202, **202**
Seated Good Morning, 123, **123**
Seated Pass to Yourself, 141, **141**
Seated Side Twist, 122, **122**

Techniques in *Four Way Burn* program (*cont.*)
  Side Bend, 169, **169**
  Side Shuffle, Drop, Clap, and Catch, 239,
      239
  Side Twist
    back problems and, 127, **127**
    in Cycle 1, 33, **33**
    golf and, 203, **203**
  Single Leg and Arm Extensions, 244, **244**
  Single-Leg Ball Passing, 243, **243**
  Single-Leg Raise and Crunch, 140, **140**
  Situp, Knee Lift, and Twist, 135, **135**
  Situp, Knee Pull, and Chop, 197, **197**
  Situp, Straight-Leg Raise, and Push, 192, **192**
  Sit Up and Pass the Ball, 136, **136**
  Sit Up and Reach, 131, **131**
  Sit Up and Reach Overhead, 187, **187**
  Soldier Walk
    in Cycle 1, 38, **38**
    cycling and, 185, **185**
    golf and, 206, **206**
    traveling and, 100, **100**
    walking and running and, 159, **159**
  Spider Walk
    in Cycle 2, 54, **54**
    golf and, 212, **212**
    walking and running and, 170, **170**
  Split Squat and Pass, 165, **165**
  Split Stand Reach to Toes
    in Cycle 3, 68, **68**
    golf and, 219, **219**
  sporting activities' benefits from, 8, 247–55
  Squat and Hold, 134, **134**
  Squat and One-Arm Reach, 157, **157**
  Squat and Push
    back problems and, 138, **138**
    in Cycle 1, 35, **35**
    cycling and, 180, **180**
    golf and, 205, **205**
  Squat and Racket Reach, 237, **237**
  Squat and Reach, 128, **128**
  Statue of Liberty
    in Cycle 2, 51, **51**
    golf and, 211, **211**

Straddle Squat and Reach
  back problems and, 133,
      133
  in Cycle 3, 61, **61**
  cycling and, 186, **186**
  golf and, 216, **216**
  traveling and, 94, **94**
Straight-Arm Toss, Hand Clap, and
    Catch, 241, **241**
Straight-Arm Toss, Side Twist, Jump,
    and Catch, 242, **242**
stretching
  Lying Side Twist, 42, **42**
  Spread Eagle, 43, **43**
  Wedge, 41, **41**
Thigh Kick and Catch
  in Cycle 1, 37, **37**
  cycling and, 181, **181**
Thigh Kick and Catch with 90-Degree-Turn
    Jumps, 172, **172**
Thigh Kick and Soldier Walk, 63, **63**
Three Way Hip, 130, **130**
tips for executing, 27, 30
Triceps and Leg Extensions
  in Cycle 4, 75, **75**
  cycling and, 193, **193**
  walking and running and, 162, **162**
Triple Jump, Back Lunge, and Side Twist, 236,
    236
Triple Jump, Forward Lunge, and Side Twist,
    233, **233**
Twist and Sweep
  back problems and, 132,
      132
  in Cycle 2, 56, **56**
  golf and, 214, **214**
  traveling and, 95, **95**
  walking and running and, 168,
      168
use of, 14, 16
Wall Squat, 124, **124**
Way Down and Way Up
  in Cycle 4, 80–81, **80–81**
  traveling and, 98, **98**

Tendons, 6

Tennis
  abdominal muscles in, 227
  ankles in, 228
  arms in, 227
  back in, 227
  feet in, 228
  fingers in, 227
  flexibility and, 228
  Four Way Burn program techniques and
    Alternating Diagonal Lunge and Reach,
      234, **234**
    benefits of, 8, 226–28
    chart, <u>245</u>
    cycles of, completing, 228–29
    Jump and Twist, 238, **238**
    Knead and Jump, 235, **235**
    overview, 228–29
    personal experience, <u>244</u>
    Pull and Chop, 230, **230**
    Quick Feet Push and Pull, 240, **240**
    Race Car Driver, 232, **232**
    Rocking Chair, 231, **231**
    Side Shuffle, Drop, Clap, and Catch, 239,
      239
    Single Leg and Arm Extensions, 244,
      244
    Single-Leg Ball Passing, 243, **243**
    Squat and Racket Reach, 237, **237**
    Straight-Arm Toss, Hand Clap, and Catch,
      241, **241**
    Straight-Arm Toss, Side Twist, Jump, and
      Catch, 242, **242**
    Triple Jump, Back Lunge, and Side Twist,
      236, **236**
    Triple Jump, Forward Lunge, and Side
      Twist, 233, **233**
  hands in, 227
  hips in, 228
  legs in, 228
  overtraining and, 7
  physical challenges of, 227–28
  professional training and, 226
  shoulders in, 227
    strength and, 228
    upper body in, 227
Thighs
  in cycling, 175–76
  in mechanics of walking and running, 148
  stretching, 90–92
Throwing activities, 247
Torso, in cycling, 175
Track and field, 254. *See also* Walking and
    running
Training, professional athletic, 10–11, 226
Trampoline, 254
Traveling
  challenges of, 87–88
  Four Way Burn program techniques and
    Around the World, 102–3, **102–3**
    chart, <u>104</u>
    Diagonal Chop, 97, **97**
    Front-Arm Raise with Leg Abduction, 96,
      96
    Golfer Swing, 99, **99**
    Good Morning with Side Twist, 93, **93**
    list of, 254
    overview, 92
    Rocking Chair, 101, **101**
    sets of, completing, 92
    Soldier Walk, 100, **100**
    Straddle Squat and Reach, 94, **94**
    Twist and Sweep, 95, **95**
    Way Down and Way Up, 98, **98**
  physical activity and, 87
  stretching and
    backs, hips, and thighs, 90–92
    neck, shoulders, and upper body, 89–90
    need for, 88–89
Tubing, rubber, 10

U

Upper body
  in cycling, 175
  in golf, 199

Upper body (*cont.*)
    in mechanics of walking and running, 148
    stretching, 89–90
    in tennis, 227

V

Vastus medialis oblique (VMO) muscle, 149,
    175–76
Volleyball, 254–55

W

Walking and running
    benefits of, 147
    buttocks muscles in, 148
    form, 150
    Four Way Burn program techniques and
        Around the World, 155, **155**
        Back Lunge Push, Pull, and Side Twist, 158,
            158
        benefits of, 8
        Carioca Loop, 163, **163**
        chart, 173
        Coil, 151–52, **151–52**
        Crossover and Reach, 156, **156**
        Front-Arm Raise with Leg Abduction, 171,
            171
        Golfer Swing, 154, **154**
        Good Morning with Side Twist, 161, **161**
        Hop and Twist, 166, **166**
        Knee Lift and Side Twist, 164, **164**
        overview, 149–51
        Pecking Bird, 160, **160**
        Rocking Chair, 167, **167**
        sessions, completing, 149–51
        Side Bend, 169, **169**
        Soldier Walk, 159, **159**
        Spider Walk, 170, **170**
        Split Squat and Pass, 165, **165**
        Squat and One-Arm Reach, 157, **157**
        Thigh Kick and Catch with 90-Degree-Turn
            Jumps, 172, **172**
        Triceps and Leg Extensions, 162, **162**
        Twist and Sweep, 168, **168**
    injury prevention, 147–48
    mechanics, 148–49
    tips, 147–48
    uneven surfaces and, 255
    weight loss and, 147
Wall technique for posture improvement, 120
Warmups, 23
Water polo, 255
Water skiing, 253
Weekend warriors, 6
Weight and back problems, 5, 118
Weight lifting and training, 11, 115–16, 250
Weight loss
    challenges of, 105
    diet and
        changes, making small, 107–8
        eating out, 111–13
        guidelines, 108–10
        low-calorie food, 112
        setpoint, finding new, 107
        shopping for food, 111
    exercise and, 15
    Four Way Burn program and, 116
    healthy, 106
    math for, 106
    personal experiences of successful, 108–9
    physical activity and, 105, 113–16, 114
    strength training and, 115–16
    walking and running and, 147
Weill, Sanford, 9
Wilkenfeld, Joel, 13
Windsurfing, 255
Wrestling, 255
Wrist weights, 21–22

Y

Yoga, 12–13